C000185445

Dr Xandria W

"Treating People – Not Cancer"

DETECTING CANCER

Gaining time: to prevent or recover from cancer

Two proposed test panels for the very early detection of cancer and guidance in non-toxic recovery strategies.

Xtra Health Publications

Book 3 in the Cancer Quintet

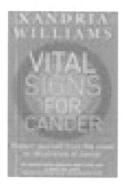

Book One

Book Two

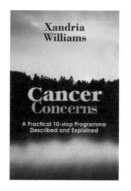

Book Three

Detecting Cancer

By

Xandria Williams

Copyright © 2013 Xandria Williams

All rights reserved. No part of this publication may be reproduced, stored in a retrieval system or transmitted in any form or by any means electronic, mechanical, audio, visual or otherwise, without prior permission of the copyright owner. Nor can it be circulated in any form of binding or cover other than that in which it is published and without similar conditions including this condition being imposed on the subsequent purchaser.

ISBN: 978-0-9568552-3-7

This book is published by Xtra Health Publications in conjunction with Writersworld Limited, and is produced entirely in the UK. It is available to order from most bookshops in the United Kingdom, and is also globally available via UK based Internet book retailers, and from the author at xandria@xandriawilliams.co.uk or Tel: 44 (0)20-7824-8153.

Copy edited by Ian Large

Cover design by Jag Lall

WRITERSWORLD
2 Bear Close Flats, Bear Close, Woodstock
Oxfordshire, OX20 1JX, England
☎ 01993 812500
☎ +44 1993 812500

www.writersworld.co.uk

The text pages of this book are produced via an independent certification process that ensures the trees from which the paper is produced come from well managed sources that exclude the risk of using illegally logged timber while leaving options to use post-consumer recycled paper as well.

ABOUT THE AUTHOR

Dr Xandria Williams, PhD, MSc, DIC, ARCS, MRSC, ND, DBM, MRN, studied chemistry at Imperial College, London and began her career as a field geochemist involved in mineral and oil exploration, working in a variety of countries in the southern hemisphere. Dr Williams was in Sydney, Australia when she changed the focus of her career and turned to biochemistry and the study of human metabolism, nutrition, naturopathy and herbal medicine. Later, she studied psychotherapy and related mental and emotional therapies such as neuro-linguistic programming (NLP) and the Emotional Freedom Technique (EFT). She has explored and used these and other methods ever since to help people with both physical health problems and emotional issues.

Dr Williams has been head of the Nutrition and Biochemistry Departments in, and lectured extensively at, several naturopathic, chiropractic and osteopathic colleges in both Australia and London. She has been a guest lecturer at colleges and events in these and other countries, and she continues to give lectures at conferences and seminars, to public interest groups and to post-graduate students.

Xandria Williams has a lucid and readily comprehensible style of lecturing and writing, even when covering complex topics. Her published works include over 400 articles and 21 books, published in several different languages, on physical and mental health care, and she has appeared frequently on radio and television.

Dr Williams has evolved her unique and highly effective approach to tackling life's physical and emotional problems over more than three decades of research, writing, teaching and helping patients. She has been in private practice for thirty years, initially in Sydney, Australia and now in Central London and County Kildare in Ireland.

Dr Xandria Williams has always helped people with a wide range of physical and emotional problems, but in recent years she has specialised in cancer and has focused progressively on researching the Cancer Process, the problems leading to it and how these can be corrected.

This book is the third in the *Cancer Quintet* series, by Xandria Williams, of which the first two are *Vital Signs for Cancer* and *Cancer Concerns*. She is currently working on Book Four, provisionally entitled *Targeting Cancer*. This series is the result of her many years as a lecturer, writer and practitioner and, specifically, of her work with people wanting to prevent, or needing to recover from, cancer.

Dr Xandria Williams sees clients at her clinics in both Central London and County Kildare, Ireland at her **CanSurvive Resource Centres.** She also works long distance with clients by phone or by Skype.

She can be contacted:

By phone on: (44) 020-7824-8153 in Central London, UK
                  (353) 046-973-1191 in Co. Kildare, Ireland

By mobile: (44) 07940-83-66-73

By email: xandria@xandriawilliams.co.uk.

Skype address: xandriaw

LinkedIn: www.linkedin.com/in/xandriawilliams.

Twitter: @XandriaWilliams

For more details see her website: www.xandriawilliams.co.uk

DISCLAIMER

This book is for information and educational purposes only and is not intended to be prescriptive or to replace appropriate professional diagnosis, guidance and help. Those concerned about cancer should seek appropriate medical, naturopathic or other appropriate health advice. In no way should anyone infer that the author claims to treat cancer. The reader is strongly advised, throughout the text, to obtain appropriate professional help for any problems that they may have.

The author and publisher have made every endeavour to ensure the accuracy of the information provided in this book. However, they assume no responsibility for unwitting errors, omissions or inaccuracies. They assume no responsibility for any inaccuracies in the source material, nor in how that material is used. The text is not intended to be comprehensive, but rather to provide general guidelines that the author considers to be of value in the maintenance of homeostasis.

More research results and evidence become available daily and many new developments may have been reported by the time this book is in print. Feel free to consult the author for further information.

OTHER BOOKS By Dr Xandria Williams INCLUDE:

Cancer Concerns	A practical 10-step programme described and explained.
Vital Signs for Cancer	Protect yourself from the onset and recurrence of cancer.
The Herbal Detox Plan	The revolutionary way to cleanse and revive your body.
Liver Detox Plan	The revolutionary way to cleanse and revive your body.
Overcoming Candida	The ultimate cookery guide.
Fatigue	The secrets of getting your energy back.
Living with Allergies	Food intolerances explained with recipes and food alternatives.
You're not Alone	A guide to understanding and overcoming feelings of isolation.
The Four Temperaments	How to achieve love, health and happiness.
From Stress to Success	10 steps to a relaxed and happy life.
Beating the Blues	A guide to avoiding and lifting depression.

Choosing Weight Intentionally How to lose weight without dieting.

What's in my Food? The nutrient content of foods in relation to their calorie content.

Choosing Health Intentionally Unlocking your subconscious for a better physical and emotional future.

How to Prevent Osteoporosis The osteoporosis diet and exercise plan.

Ideal Weight Ideal Shape

Building Stronger Bones Naturally

Nutritional Supplements formulated by Dr Xandria Williams:

Liver Support

Adrenomax

Books and supplements are available from Dr Xandria Williams:

By phone on: (44) 020-7824-8153 (UK) or (353) 046-973-1191 (Ireland)

By email: xandria@xandriawilliams.co.uk.

The supplements are also available from Nutri Advanced on 0-800-212-742 or 44 (0)-1663-718-804.

ACKNOWLEDGEMENTS

It is inevitable that, after forty years in this profession, I owe thanks to more people than I can name, count or list. I would, however, like to offer thanks to the following, and I ask those that I have not mentioned specifically to accept my thanks as well. They know who they are.

Lecturing: My start in this profession was due to the persuasion of the then Head of the Sydney College of Chiropractic who needed a biochemistry teacher and persuaded me to face an audience. Initially nervous, I soon came to love it. This was quickly followed by long-term lectureships at several other natural therapies colleges, in both Australia and the UK, over the next forty years, mainly in biochemistry and nutritional therapeutics, but occasionally in other related subjects. This lecturing gave me the incentive to explore and organise all I have learnt in, and related to, the field of natural medicine and alternative and complementary therapies. The countless organisations and interest groups that have asked for individual lectures and seminars have focused my attention on covering the topics for people with a wide range and levels of backgrounds and interests.

Writing: My thanks go to a number of publishers by whom I have been asked to write over 400 articles. In particular I would like to thank Russell Atkinson of *Nature and Health Journal* who was the first to persuade me I could write as well as talk, and Barbara McGregor of *Australian Wellbeing*, plus editors of many other journals. These include *Prevention Magazine* and *Discover Better Health* in Australia, and *Here's Health* and *Good Health* in the UK. Thanks are due to Patrick Gallagher of Allen and Unwin Australia for convincing and persuading me that I could make the stretch from articles to books, and to the many publishers that have since endorsed this: Nature and Health Books, Simon and Schuster, Letts Publishing, Cedar, Hodder and Stoughton, Time-Life Books, Element Books, Vermillion, Thorsons, Hamlyn, Piatkus, North Atlantic Books and Xtra Health Publications, plus many in foreign languages. These have helped me spread the information about the natural therapies to a far wider audience than I could have done on my own. Special thanks are due to my agent and good friend Sara Menguc who has supported the writing and publication of all but my first few books.

Colleagues and clients: Many dozens of colleagues have been inspiring sharers of knowledge and with them I have enjoyed many vital, happy, interesting, challenging and productive discussions. The same can be said for the many thousands of students with whom I have had the privilege to share information and who have attended my lectures, seminars and workshops. I particularly wish to thank the many thousands of patients who have entrusted me with their problems, provided me with countless opportunities to learn so much more about health and emotional issues, and shared with me so many positive outcomes.

In relation to the test panels described in this book in particular I would like to thank Dr Emil Schandl of American Metabolic Laboratories in the US, and Dr Olga Galkina of The Galkina Laboratory in the UK. They both, in their unique ways, provided me with the starting points for the research that led to the thesis that forms Section II of this book, and helped me in my exploration of these topics. By providing, in their respective laboratories, the tests referred to here they have enabled me, and many other health care professionals working in this field, to help a wide variety of people. Long may their work and services continue.

On a personal note I would like to acknowledge the prompting of my long-term friend, Dr Timothy Moulton, Professor of Ecology at the Universidade do Estado do Rio de Janeiro who convinced me that my work merited presentation for a doctorate. Finally I deeply acknowledge and am grateful for the love, help and support of my aunt Shelagh Riall, nee Williams, whom I met when eighteen, and who I described in my book *Stress Recognise and Resolve* as 'my aunt, my friend, my guide and my inspiration'. She is sorely missed.

DEDICATION

From the original Hippocratic Oath:

*"I will prescribe regimens for the good of my patients according to my ability and my judgment and **never do harm** to anyone."*

This is commonly translated by many as
"First do no harm".

This book is dedicated to people who are aware of and concerned about the escalating increase in the incidence of cancer over recent years and the limited success that results from drugs, radiation and surgery, and are conscious of the significant harm that can be done by such treatments. These people include those who are developing the many tests described here, and those who are researching and developing the many helpful and non-toxic alternative remedies that can be used by those who wish to avoid harmful treatments.

It is dedicated to the individuals who are keen to explore other options and rational methods of cancer prevention and treatment that are in harmony with their bodies, and who also require a strong evidence base for the benefits of the suggestions made to them. It is dedicated to all those who recognise the wisdom of their body as a potentially self-maintaining and self-healing entity, provided its nutrient and other needs are met and it is spared the onslaught of avoidable toxins and other damaging agents and lifestyle habits.

It is dedicated to all people who are working hard to prevent cancer, in themselves and others, by rational and natural means, to people who care for those with cancer and to people who have cancer and are looking to take some personal responsibility for their care and their future, and who have the commitment and discipline to follow through on the many lifestyle changes that are required for the harmonious recovery of optimum health without adverse and toxic side effects.

PREFACE

Detecting Cancer is a tour de force that could change the world. I write that huge statement because the science behind the tests outlined in Xandria Williams' new book, the third in the series, is not only sound and well evidenced but, used collectively, is totally cutting edge, effective and will save lives at a time when the trend for cancers is increasing steadily worldwide.

In Great Britain, for example, the age-standardised incident rates for all cancers increased by 2% for males and by 6% for females during the last ten years, with a sad slowing down of the previous trend of decreasing cancer mortalities from the early '90s. Today, more than 300,000 people are newly diagnosed each year. These rates of cancer represented 28% of all deaths in the UK in 2010, over 77,000 <u>more</u> cancer deaths than from heart disease and nearly 110,000 more cancer deaths than those from stroke. Nearly 160,000 individuals, beloved by their family and friends, died in 2010 of this insidious condition and became part of these statistics (Figure 1). Their time had come.

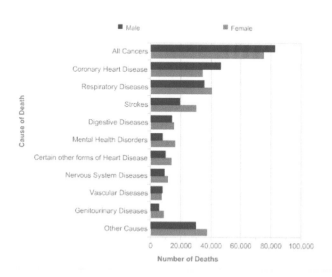

Figure 1. The Ten Most Common Causes of Death, Numbers of Death per Year, Ages one and over, UK 2010.

Cancer Research UK, who publish this information, tell us in their policy statement[1] that the *"early detection of cancer is critical to its successful treatment. At present, around 45% of patients are diagnosed at a stage when cancer can be successfully treated. Earlier diagnosis is likely to have an impact on cancer mortality, although this varies from cancer to cancer, and is more achievable in some cancers than others."*

Early diagnosis is EXACTLY what this brave, ground-breaking book is about. Using non-invasive tests, Dr Williams tells us how researchers have shown that certain substances produced by the body will invariably change as cancer gets worse and then change again as the body fights it, as it can be empowered to do. Well, we've heard that before… except we haven't, not quite. Because these are substances the vast majority of health workers in cancer care will not have even heard of yet. They will, in time, but you can read about them here, now. But what's even more interesting, is that these substances are produced, in many circumstances, BEFORE any tumour is large enough to be detected by conventional methods. Which means using the combined results of these tests gives us very early detection of cancer, very much earlier than is conventionally possible at the moment, and with no cutting, squashing or loud magnetic banging! Early enough in fact, that with any Red Alert from these tests, substantial changes in diet and lifestyle, together with individually prescribed supplements for that particular person's metabolism, will bring about the necessary biochemical and other changes for the body to return to homeostasis, or healthy balance. The process towards cancer is stopped. Detectable by these tests, those changes will provide a visual changing trend of those potentially worrying components. And then keep them down. And that means no cancer. That would be called a cure in most languages except it's achieved without invasive surgery, without the cancer risk factors of radiation and without the toxicity of chemotherapy. But still a cure.

Of course, in some cases sadly, these tests will confirm what is already known. That a cancer is present in amounts detectable conventionally. In this situation, these combination tests that Dr

---

[1] www.cancerresearchuk.org/cancer-info/publicpolicy/ourpolicypositions/ symptom_Awareness

Williams outlines can be used to ensure that recommended medical treatment options are working, that it is the right protocol to help that particular individual, rather than just 'The Treatment for that particular Type of Cancer'. The patient may wish to support and supplement their conventional medical treatment. This can be done using the scientifically-grounded wisdom and knowledge in the evidence-based work Williams presented in her previous books, *Vital Signs for Cancer* and *Cancer Concerns.* Thus, with the focus on the person (the patient) rather than on the disease, the information in *Cancer Concerns* would provide a practical ten-step programme. Working individually is the way forward and the way forward is these tests. And these tests show it and show when it's there and when it's not, whether things work and also when they don't.

The author comes from that small group of contrarians who dares to question whether what is available right now, in medical cancer testing, is good enough. For the attainment of her PhD Doctorate award, she showed therein that the principles of such an award are still rightly reflective of the 'love of wisdom'. This passion for knowledge and for sharing it with us all has been shown in her many other books. For the past decade, her passion has extended to researching and helping people with cancer. It has made her realise and propose therefore both within her thesis and wherever folk will listen, that cancer actually is not the disease we've heard so much about. It is, in fact, a process, actually starting ages before that ghastly frightening tumour is detectable. One doesn't suddenly wake up one morning 'with' cancer; it's been creeping up inexorably for ages, often years. However, arguably within six weeks of commencement of that process, it is now detectable by these tests that she describes. Even if the process might take eight years to result in the detectable disease we call cancer.

Xandria Williams was not involved in the development of the tests she describes but she has brought them together, has built them into a coherent concept, has explained them and the foundation for them, and is spreading the word. The tests were developed by other wonderful scientists and doctors throughout the world committed to pushing the boundaries of scientific research just that little bit further. Sometimes, over decades. This dedicated research is done to benefit humanity yet we are all increasingly seeing cancer deaths rise – despite any political so-called 'War on Cancer'. The work of these scientists is individually regarded as Gold Standard science – evidence-based research, published and peer reviewed; yet sometimes they just stay that way and the research doesn't get out there!

The tests are not invasive as are some others, indeed most other tests. For what they are, they are also relatively inexpensive; certainly compared to many other forms of screening. These blood- or urine-based tests are totally unlike those currently used for diagnosing this most dreaded condition or, indeed, for monitoring the progress of any form of cancer treatment. Yet they could and should be widely used not only for very early diagnosis but also for ensuring the treatments chosen are on track and working effectively.

This very well-referenced book is not for the faint hearted. Nor does it appear to be an easy read for many of us, being the most complex of her current trilogy. But don't worry; she recognises that and presents us with a choice – we can dive in or dip in, go as deep or as shallow as we wish, with the right amount of information and/or science as we want or can handle at any one time. Because Dr Xandria Williams is a naturopathic physician and a biochemist, yet also trained in psychotherapy, she understands what makes us tick. She knows that if we are worried about cancer, we're unlikely to be able to handle too much, too soon; we need short bites and it needs to make sense, fast. Then, when we start beginning to understand there's something we can actually do that empowers us by bringing us information about our charting of our own recovery, then we can handle and understand the extra deeper levels of information; however complex they may at first appear in the book.

Interestingly, whilst not denying great work is undertaken bringing grateful praise and thanks from many, the published objective and ambition of Cancer Research is 'to bring forward the day when all cancers are cured'. This is interesting as one might have hoped we would prefer to look forward to the *prevention* of cancer, not purely its cure. It must be the higher goal. But there's a lot at stake of course. As the biggest single independent funder of cancer research throughout Europe if not the world, supporting the work of more than

4,000 scientists, doctors and nurses across the UK, with over 35,000 employees and 40,000 volunteers, what would all those folk do if cancer actually could be prevented?

These tests will not prevent cancer. But their use might prevent the acceleration of the process in each individual that *causes* cancer by increasing understanding of what's happening in each of our bodies. I hope Dr Williams' thesis in this book will be read widely by anyone concerned by cancer and especially by Cancer Research UK. To get their mighty weight behind this so these tests become extensively used and properly on the map would do more good than has probably occurred in cancer research for far too long. But *Detecting Cancer* is not written for an organisation; its message is too important to run the risk of getting overlooked, side-lined and covered in cobwebs; as has so much brilliant research in the past. The wheel gets constantly re-invented.

This book has been written from the passion which Dr Williams ND, PhD, holds for helping folk with cancer concerns to understand what's been happening, at cellular level, how to detect it, how to track it and what to do about it. And it works. This book could quite possibly save your life.

Chris Burley ND, MRN, Naturopathic Physician
Immediate Past President, General Council and Register of
Naturopaths, October 2013

––––––––––––––––––

Cancer is a growing problem and is expected to escalate worldwide for years to come due to our toxic environment and lack of education as to the healthiest lifestyles and choices people can make in their life. For people who want to explore alternative options on their own, or in combination with conventional medication, commonly referred to as integrative medicine, there is an abundance of extensively researched and proven information. However, this very abundance poses a problem. Who should you believe? What course should you follow? What is the evidence? You will find thoroughly researched and knowledgeably designed approaches for detection and testing contained within this book.

Dr Xandria Williams has degrees in chemistry and a solid foundation of biochemistry, particularly as it relates to cancer. Her medical training in alternative medicine as a naturopath in Australia and her thirty years of practical experience with patients gives her a wealth of experience on which her writing is based. In the last ten years she has focused on and researched the biochemical underpinnings of the alternative approaches to cancer and helped many people with the problem. All this is evidenced in the depth of material that she presents in this book and her confidence in the concepts she describes and explains.

It is known by many authorities in the field of medicine who do not have a financially vested interest in cancer detection, such as in mammograms and other cancer testing, that these tests are not extremely accurate in many instances and may even give false readings. Nor do they constitute truly early warning signs. To do just one of the conventionally recommended tests for cancer can be very limiting as to identifying the status or existence of a cancer and whether it be early detection or later diagnosis of cancer needs to be verified by more extensive testing. In this, Dr Williams' third book in her series on cancer, she focuses on the extent and approaches to testing that can be done to determine firstly whether or not you have cancer and secondly, and very importantly, what you can do about it. She provides ample evidence, confirmed by the research literature, that the use of the results of her selected tests forms a valid basis for both assessing the situation and planning a recovery.

It is a pleasure to write this preface to her latest book and we wish you, her readers, success in your endeavours to initially prevent and thereby avoid cancer altogether or to have the tools and information to make wise and educated decisions as to the course of treatment you might choose. This book compiles well-researched and documented knowledge and expertise that can possibly help change the direction and longevity of your life. If you want to try alternative or complementary options and your doctors tell you they are unproven, give them this book. It is fully referenced to academic research papers that very clearly are proven.

Dr Mark Dargan Smith
Chairman of the Board, Chancellor and Dean
University of Natural Medicine, USA

The human body is designed to heal itself. In fact, it is so good at repairing itself that we take it for granted. Most of us only recognise a health problem as a medical condition if the body isn't able to recover on its own.

Our immune system can activate quickly and handle things like the common cold. However, there are illnesses and underlying processes that we can't see or feel that sometimes evade or overpower the immune system that can cause permanent damage to our body over long periods of time.

If we had a way to uncover the biochemical changes that are happening deep within our body before the process had caused permanent damage or irreversible illness we would have much greater odds of preventing that damage. These are what I call reversible health challenges or illnesses.

This is exactly what Dr Xandria Williams is proposing in her new book, *Detecting Cancer*, before it has devastated the body beyond its ability to repair itself. None of us want to hear our doctor tell us we have cancer. But for the most part we don't do anything, often out of our ignorance, until we are faced with the 'You have Cancer' diagnosis.

What Dr Williams has uncovered and brought together are revolutionary biochemical tests that have the potential to predict or uncover subtle changes that are taking place within our body's chemistry. Her work is based on her lifetime of experience in providing nutritional and lifestyle coaching to thousands of clients and at the same time evaluating visual, physical and biochemical changes (individually and in combinations) that are occurring within the body that others have missed, overlooked, or not even sought.

I think it's time that we look at what she is proposing with open eyes and ears. The old paradigm promoted by most of the traditional medical community of not worrying until real symptoms are evident and confirmed by a very limited set of tests is not working. Preventive health or, if a problem is identified, restoring health, is fundamentally different than treating symptoms.

I encourage every layperson and everyone involved in all the medical professions to look at what Xandria Williams is proposing as a new way of detecting subtle biochemical changes before we reach the point of no return. At the least it can't hurt you and at the best it might save your life or one of your loved ones. If the news is not good, she then offers you the benefit of tests that provide information that can help you to recover without causing further damage.

This book should be in everyone's hands. Get an extra copy and share it with your friends. And thanks Xandria for being one of the pioneers in the natural health movement.

Dr Larry Milam
President
University of Natural Medicine, USA

COMMENT

I was diagnosed with an Advanced Stage Prostate Cancer in 2002 following the usual procedures of biopsy, blood tests and scans. The result was my choosing to have the Radical Prostatectomy operation in July of that year, when a large tumour was removed.

A period of recovery was followed by blood tests, which indicated my PSA slowly rising. MRI, Bone and CT scans followed and my consultants advised Radical Radiotherapy Treatment, Monday to Friday, over a five-week period. I followed their advice and completed this treatment.

I first met Xandria Williams in 2001. I was a patient with a swollen tummy, which Xandria immediately diagnosed as an allergy. In between taking advantage of her advice on my particular problem, I heard her speak in clear and logical fashion on the value of healthy eating and alternative medicines and her special application to cancer.

With my cancer, I went straight to Xandria for professional support and advice on a recovery programme. Xandria explained how detailed tests would provide information from which the most exact and appropriate programme could be selected for my individual needs. This was the CA Profile of which I am still taking advantage. My condition has benefitted from Xandria's particular expertise and exceptional professional knowledge. The results have improved in the years since, and the positive results shown on my latest CA Profile test are proven testament to Xandria's guidance and the development of her work.

David Pearson
October 2013

TABLE OF CONTENTS

SECTION II - THESIS

The very early detection of cancer.
Two proposed test panels for early detection and planning a recovery programme.

PRELIMINARIES

CHAPTER 1

INTRODUCTION

This is a book in two parts.

Section I is a descriptive section covering the tests that are proposed for what is thought to be the earliest possible detection of cancer and for a sound basis on which to base a recovery plan.

Section II is a technical description of the same material, in the form of a PhD thesis and contains the references to the statements made.

<u>**Section I**</u> is for the general reader. It includes a brief introduction to cancer. This is followed by a description of the way your cells function and the way cancer develops. Based on this knowledge there is a description of the two proposed Test Panels.

The 'Early Warning' First Test Panel is useful if you want to know:

* whether or not you have cancer, even before a tumour can be detected;
* whether or not, if you have had cancer, any treatments have been successful;
* if you are in remission or if cancer has returned, even in a very minor way.

The Second Test Panel is useful if you have cancer and want to learn more about its unique characteristics and to determine the best way to deal with it and what natural remedies or nutrients to use to restore your body to homeostasis[2] and health. The results of the tests that make up this panel can both warn you of impending problems and help you plan a recovery programme.

---

[2] Homeostasis: the tendency of the body to maintain internal stability, owing to the coordinated response of its parts to any situation or stimulus that would alter its normal condition or function.

Time to Recover

This information, properly used, will give you 'time to recover', either from a fully developed, tumour-based diagnosis of cancer, or from the earliest indications that you may be starting along the Cancer Process but with, as yet, no identifiable tumour. Inevitably, the sooner you start on corrections the easier it is to recover.

In the interest of easy reading and the flow of information, the statements in Section I are not referenced, but if you want further information on any statements made you will find supportive references and the evidence behind the statements in Section II.

Section II is a technical thesis covering the research basis and the evidence that lies behind the proposed tests. It is technical and well referenced.

You may or may not want to read the level of detail found in Section II for yourself. However, if you are interested in the complementary, alternative and metabolic (CAM) or naturopathic methods for both detecting and describing the unique characteristics of an individual's cancer, this book can offer you many benefits. At the end of Section II you will find some case histories that demonstrate the use and value of these tests. I recommend that you read them, even if you skip much of Section II.

If you are concerned about, or have, cancer, and want to incorporate CAM methods into what you do on your road to recovery, either wholly or in part, you may well face opposition. You will almost certainly be faced with at least some people who try to talk you out of this. They will, all too often, try to discourage you from taking the initiative. Instead they may well encourage you to follow the medical model of surgery, chemotherapy or radiation, trying to convince you that not following the medical, drug and surgery (MDS) approach is foolhardy. They may mean well, but they may not be aware of either (a) the harm the MDS system can do and the limited benefit it offers, long term; or (b) the benefits that can come from the CAM approach and that are achieved without toxic or harmful effects in either the short or long term.

These people may include members of your family, friends, colleagues, employers or people you may meet more casually. It may also include your medical team, and in fact will almost certainly do so. They may say that CAM methods do not work. They may say that there is no proof or evidence for any benefit of what you are doing or proposing to do. This is not true.

If you have already read the first two books in this series you will know that there is, in fact, a large and significant amount of referenced research that validates the CAM approaches to cancer. This book takes that evidence base further. It can be useful for you to show to your doctors if they insist there is no proof for anything you may be doing that is deemed 'alternative' or 'complementary'. It may also be helpful, again as validation of what you are doing, when family, friends, colleagues or employers try to argue you out of what you are doing.

Overview

Cancer is so feared that many people prefer to put their head in the sand and ignore the possibility that they may be developing it. For this reason it is important to keep emphasising the point that cancer is a degenerative disease that can be prevented or managed, just as can diabetes. It can be managed in ways that are non toxic, do not cause adverse side or toxic effects, do not make your hair fall out, do not make you feel ill, rotten, nauseous or lacking in energy, and do not compromise your health as an 'acceptable' side effect. In fact the reverse is true. When you learn to manage your lifestyle and diet correctly you will almost certainly feel an enormous improvement in overall health and wellbeing and a boost in energy.

Cancer can be prevented or managed by:

a) removing or minimising the Predisposing Factors in your life;
b) doing the tests to make sure you remain clear of the start of the Cancer Process;
c) correcting the results of the tests, if they are found to be outside the normal range;
d) altering your lifestyle to one that supports you in restoring good health.

You almost certainly follow this procedure, or you should, for your car. Do it for yourself. You can replace your car. You cannot replace yourself.

Can you 'cure' cancer, to the extent that you can stop being concerned about it? No, but in the same sense you cannot 'cure' hunger or thirst. You can 'manage' hunger and thirst, temporarily. You eat. You drink. But if, once satisfied, you then stop eating and drinking you will, some hours later, find that the symptoms have returned; you will feel hunger and thirst again. The problem will return. You can 'manage' hunger and thirst by adjusting your lifestyle so that you eat and drink at regular intervals, as appropriate. In the same way you can 'manage' cancer, both its prevention and your recovery from it, by taking the appropriate action in relation to your diet and lifestyle.

There is now a large body of research that attributes the cause of cancer to external factors, not to your genes, but to your lifestyle, including your diet, and to other factors over which, to a large extent, you can exert some control. Many researchers now put this figure as high as 93% to 95%.

This will be fully demonstrated as you read through the following pages.

You will learn many important things from this book, and it is appropriate to outline them briefly here.

- You will learn that cancer is largely a disease of your chosen lifestyle, including your diet. In fact it can be as much as 93 per cent, arguably even more, due to errors of lifestyle.
- You make daily decisions about your lifestyle. This means that, daily, you can have a major control over whether or not you get cancer, and, if cancer has started, whether or not you recover from it.
- Many people know some of the things that they are doing that are bad for their health, and things they should be doing that would improve their health, but they need a nudge or a trigger,

possibly the early warning of cancer, before they are willing to make such changes. Perhaps you are one of these people.

- If you are unwilling to make any changes in your lifestyle until it becomes a matter of urgency, the sooner you can detect cancer and get the required nudge to improve your lifestyle, the greater is your chance of either prevention or recovery.

- Cancer, usually in the form of a tumour, does not start suddenly. Cancer is process, a two-part process.

- In Phase One you do not have cancer. You do, however, have a number of Predisposing Factors. These are touched on below and discussed more fully in Book One of this *Cancer Quintet*, entitled *Vital Signs for Cancer*. These Predisposing Factors include poor diet and nutrient deficiencies, an overload of toxins, and a progression of health problems, from adrenal exhaustion, to diabetes, accompanied by unresolved or excessive stresses that are not properly managed.

- In Phase Two you do have cancer. You have finally developed some cells, cells that behave differently to normal healthy cells, cells that are out of control and can multiply without the usual restraints, and thus, eventually, build up into a detectable tumour. Further, they have the ability to migrate and form new tumours elsewhere, to metastasise; and this is the real danger of malignant cancer.

- To the extent that you are in control of your lifestyle, and this is almost certainly a greater extent than you may think, you can do a great deal to reverse this Cancer Process whenever you choose.

- You will learn in the following pages that you can detect the very earliest start of the Cancer Process, at a time when recovery is very much easier than it would be if you waited until a detectable tumour had formed.

- Some people are afraid to do such tests, thinking that, if the results are bad, their only options will be surgery, chemotherapy or radiation. But doing these tests and modifying your lifestyle may, in fact, mean that you can pull back and actually avoid having to follow, or be subjected to any of these three strategies.

- You will learn that there is a group of tests, based on a single blood sample; the proposed early warning 'First Test Panel', the results of which can alert you to the presence of active cancer cells as soon as six weeks after the first cancer cells form. This one test panel covers the possibility of cancer anywhere in your whole body. There is no need to do separate tests for breast, lung, liver, colon, prostate or cancer at any other specific location. This one panel of tests will do it all.

- Cancer is a systemic problem. It is not a local problem, at least initially. As such, a recovery plan should be systemic, involving lifestyle changes and working harmoniously with your body. It should not involve drugs and harmful or unpleasant treatments. There should be no harsh treatment, no treatment that damages other aspects of yourself. Thus there is little to fear from following such a corrective regime, and much to be gained by it, for not only the prevention of cancer or the recovery from it, but for your overall health and wellbeing.

- The results from this First Test Panel, if they are abnormal, while they cover your overall system, will not tell you where a possible cancer is located, or is likely to develop. That would matter in a tumour-focused approach to treatment which is aimed almost entirely at tumour destruction, no matter the collateral damage or cost to the rest of your body, and with little thought as to why and how it developed. This is the approach adopted by the medical profession. Knowing where a tumour might develop is much less important than detecting and correcting the systemic errors that are present and thus preventing cancer or reversing the Cancer Process. This is the CAM or naturopathic approach. It is the whole-body approach where it is the person that is treated, not the tumour, where the aim is to restore homeostasis or normal and healthy function.

- You will learn that there is a second group of tests, the proposed 'Second Test Panel'. The information derived from the results of this Second Test Panel will enhance the information derived from the First Test Panel. If the first group of results was marginal, the results of this Second Test Panel will help to resolve any ambiguity.

- More importantly, the results of this Second Test Panel will provide information as to the nature of the developing cancer, its strengths and its weaknesses. They can be used to plan and target your recovery and return you to good health. This means that instead of doing or taking everything that you are told about or read about that 'will help you fight cancer', you can refine and target your approach. You can avoid the less successful shotgun approach. You can save time, money and effort and have a greater chance of success.

- You will learn, and may be surprised to know, that there is an immense body of research that backs up and supports the use of these two panels of tests. This is elaborated in the thesis that makes up Section II of this book. This thesis is fully referenced and you can search for yourself each of the research papers if you wish to be even surer of the basis for these concepts. You can also put the appropriate words into a search engine and learn more, or obtain reinforcement for the ideas expressed here.

The layout of this book is somewhat unusual. It encompasses a first half that is for the general reader. It includes some general discussions as to the nature of your body, its cells, and the way cancer develops. It then gives a general description of the two test panels and how the results can be used. The second half is a thesis that covers the research foundation for the two test panels. This part may not interest the general reader but does provide a solid foundation to the proposed tests. At the end of it there are several useful and very different case histories. This latter part should certainly be of interest, use and value to your practitioners or medical team, who may well not be aware of much of this material.

Ideally, if you want to follow this approach to cancer, you should find a practitioner who is happy to work with you along these lines. Cancer is much too big a problem for you to handle without help, in fact for anyone to handle without help. You will also need a practitioner to organise the tests for you.

You can follow a number of options. You can read this Introduction and then look for a professional who can help you. You can read this

Introduction, then Section I and the Case Histories from Section II, and then find a practitioner who will help you with the tests. For further information, and particularly if you already have some understanding of cancer, you can explore Section II, either skimming over the more technical details, or delving into it more deeply. For you to feel confident in the tests and to understand their usefulness it is not necessary for you to understand the full science of the thesis, but if you skim over it and get the general picture you will be reassured as to the foundation for the ideas expressed here.

You can also use this book when faced with the doubters, those that would have you ignore all alternative options, wait until a tumour is fully formed, and succumb to the big three: surgery, chemotherapy and radiation.

* If the CAM or naturopathic route to cancer recovery appeals to you but your doctor or oncologist is not supportive and is telling you the ideas are unproven or not evidence-based, and if you want their support, use this book. Give it to your medical team and show them the second half, Section II, with all its information and the several hundred references to research studies. If they refuse to look at it or read it you may want to consider whether or not you are receiving the best care, or the care that is consistent with your own goals for yourself. It is your life.

* If your family or friends are trying to persuade you away from it, you could also pass this book on to them. If they read it they may become more supportive of your chosen path to recovery.

* If you are looking for a practitioner to help you work in this way, then giving them this book, and discussing this approach, will help you in your choice of practitioner. If you already have a practitioner, you may want to give this book to them to ensure that you and they are working together.

That is a brief overview or summary of this book. The various points will be picked up and discussed as we go along.

Before we fully begin it is also important to think about time. If or when cancer is once diagnosed, most people find that they are being rushed, in many ways. They are being rushed into coming to terms with what is often a terrifying and overwhelming diagnosis, and they are being rushed into making decisions on the basis of too little knowledge, and following treatments they may later come to regret. They may also be made to feel powerless about their own ability to do anything to aid their recovery. So let us consider time, in this context.

CHAPTER 2

TIME TO RECOVER

The fundamental message of *Detecting Cancer*, subtitled *Gaining time: to prevent or recover from cancer*, is simple and is described here, in its overall concept. There are several key facts to take from this, all of which are fully explained and validated in the following pages.

Time

In this book you will learn many factors about cancer that you may not have thought about. Some have already been touched on. They are grouped together here for reinforcement and clarity:

- Cancer can take a long time to develop, and yours, if you already have cancer, has probably taken many months and possibly even years to reach the stage at which it has been detected.

- Thus, when you are finally diagnosed with cancer you have probably had it for a long time.

- This in turn means that you do not necessarily need to rush into treatments, certainly not into ones that come with toxic and often irreversible side effects, the moment cancer is discovered. Your doctor or specialists may recommend this and may try to impress on you the need for immediate and rapid action. They may insist there is not sufficient time for you to go away and think, to read up, and to consider your options. However, there is little evidence that taking time, a few days certainly, weeks possibly, to research your options is going to worsen your outcome. It may even improve your outcome as your research may show you some of the pitfalls of the first chosen treatment or treatments and the benefits of some other options that you discover during this time.

- It is important that you take the time to do the various tests described here, tests that will help you to target the specific aspects of your particular cancer, not only as to its location but as to its unique characteristics; characteristics that can lead to a targeted and positive recovery plan.

- Cancer is largely, though of course not entirely, a disease of the last hundred years and is overwhelmingly due to errors in your lifestyle, including your diet.

- Cancer is not the result of faulty genes that you were born with. You are not your genes. No matter what genes you are born with, cancer is not inevitable. Cancer is the result of cellular changes, caused by external or epigenetic (outside your genes) agents. These epigenetic agents from your diet and lifestyle trigger cellular changes which in turn activate a number of inactive genes. These inactive genes, called pro-oncogenes, once activated, become oncogenes and can cause cancer. But note they only become dangerous oncogenes when activated by these initiating cellular faults, which in turn are triggered by your lifestyle.

- You may be surprised to discover that this has been known since 1925, that it was stated by Nobel Prize winner Dr Otto Warburg, and that this view continues to be supported and validated by current research.

- Based on this understanding, it is clearly important that you take the time to learn all you can about both your lifestyle errors and the ways in which you can make improvements.

- The test panels described here, and their results, can give you the information and the time.

- Your recovery protocol will take time. Cancer is a serious problem and its reversal or eradication demands a serious input from you. Many of the actions you can take to improve your lifestyle do demand, at least at first, the allocation of time.

- It can also be argued that for many people it becomes appropriate to treat cancer as a disease that can be managed, in a manner somewhat similar to diabetes, and that for as long as you maintain the appropriate and healthy lifestyle, you can remain free from its damaging consequences.

- You need to allow yourself the time and space to achieve this recovery or managed state.

- If you take all the necessary steps you will recover, or return to homeostasis, certainly for a lot longer than if you continue to follow your present lifestyle.

- If you don't yet have a cancer diagnosis but are concerned that you may have cancer, or if you want to do all you can to prevent it, doing the tests described here can give you both the information and the time to avoid the development of cancer.

To Recover

- The First Test Panel, based on a blood and a urine sample, can detect cancer as early as six weeks after the formation of the first cancer cells, and as much as fourteen years before a tumour can be detected.[3]

- The method of collecting the sample and the laboratory to which it can be submitted are explained in Section I.

- If your results from the First Test Panel are normal you can be reasonably sure that you have not started along the Cancer Process and that you are unlikely to develop or be diagnosed with cancer in the next few years.

- If the results of this early First Test Panel suggest that you have started along the Cancer Process, along the path of cellular changes that could lead to a tumour, then it is time to take stock and to make changes in your lifestyle. These changes are discussed in the first two books in this *Cancer Quintet* series: *Vital Signs for Cancer* and *Cancer Concerns*.

- If any one of your results of the First Test Panel is outside the normal range, cancer is a possibility, though not assured. However, since the CAM approaches to restoring homeostasis are harmless and non toxic, and since they all contribute to improved health overall, and to the avoidance of a number of other degenerative diseases, you would be well advised to start making some positive changes in your lifestyle right away. You would also be well advised to do a repeat test three

---

[3] Dr E. Schandl, American Metabolic Laboratories.

months later to make sure there has been (a) an improvement or (b) no worsening of your situation.

- If more than one result from the First Test Panel is outside the normal range, now is the time to start a more serious Recovery Plan. Don't delay. This early detection can help you to reverse out of the Cancer Process. Delay will allow the process to proceed and your health to deteriorate. Correction becomes increasingly difficult as cancer develops.

- The Second Test Panel is a set of tests that is recommended if the First Test Panel shows errors indicative of an active Cancer Process. The results will show the specific aspects of your cancer development that need to be corrected. This in turn will allow a more targeted and successful Recovery Plan to be designed for you.

- The details of both test panels are given below, in brief and in general outline, and in detail in Section II.

- You may have been told that cancer is the result of your genes and that there is little you can do about it. To a large extent this is not true. As Dr Otto Warburg demonstrated, in 1925, cancer is the result of cellular changes that in turn can 'turn-on' or damage proto-oncogenes. Proto-oncogenes are the genes that are inactive until an external trigger activates them or 'turns them on'. These altered genes then become fully developed and active oncogenes. Oncogenes are ones that stimulate the development of cancer. They can lead to the cellular changes that become overt and fully-developed cancer. This may seem to be an extraordinary sequence of events, of no use and with immense potential harm. However, as you will discover, the action of many of these activated proto-oncogenes does offer some benefits, mostly during embryonic life, or in certain times of recovery. An example of the former is the activation of CEA (see below in the First Test Panel) and the latter includes increased capillary growth or angiogenesis when it is needed for wound healing (discussed as part of the Second Test Panel).

- It is important to understand that the original causes of cancer are the epigenetic (literally 'outside your genes', in fact usually outside your body) factors that cause the early cellular changes, and that these triggers come, necessarily, from a bad diet and a poor lifestyle, in all its many manifestations.

- This last point is incredibly powerful. You are, to a large extent, in control of your diet and much of your lifestyle. You can avoid or minimise the harm to which you may be exposed. This means you can be in control of (a) early detection; (b) orchestrating your recovery; and (c) the whole process that is aimed at restoring homeostasis (the normal function of your body) and that the Recovery Process is both non-toxic and can improve your overall health, wellbeing and longevity as well as your recovery from cancer.

SECTION I

CHAPTER 3

CANCER AND YOUR CELLS

To understand the reasons for the tests and the implications of the results of these tests it is important to understand how cancer develops. To do this you need to know more about your cells. So we will start by discussing the cell with its surrounding membrane, which is hugely important, and several of the internal organelles (think of the organs within your whole body), including the mitochondria, the ribosomes (briefly) and the nucleus. Inside the nucleus we will find the genes and learn more about the role they play in cancer, although you will probably find that this role is more limited than you may have assumed. We will also need to consider the enzymes (biological catalysts) that are made according to the dictates of your genes.

Once this foundation is laid we will explore the concept of cancer as an evolving process, rather than simply the presence of a tumour, and find out how it starts and then develops. This will involve a discussion of mitochondrial failure, stem cells and the external or epigenetic factors that are part of your lifestyle, including, but not limited to your diet.

You will gradually take on board the power of the concept that by far the most important causes of cancer, the initial triggering factors, are not your genes, but aspects of your lifestyle and the empowering concept that you are, to a large extent, in control of your lifestyle. Thus you can have a major input into preventing cancer and, if required, in orchestrating your recovery.

I make no apology for the increasing technical detail provided here, or for the use of repetition to help carry the understanding forward and enhance the flow of the topic. I hope I have written it in such a way that if you skim over the sentences that are too complex you will come to an oasis of descriptive calm such that you can pick up the story and get the general gist of what is being described and can make use of it. Please understand that this series of books is aimed at students and at practitioners who have not yet specialised in cancer, as well as at the general reader and people dealing with their own, or someone else's cancer.

Your Cells

The following information is fundamental to an understanding of the way in which cancer develops. The description is basic and simplified. The full scenario is very much more complicated. However, this description will serve our needs and these concepts will give you a working idea of what to test for and then, based on the results of these tests, what to consider incorporating into a Recovery Protocol.

The important parts of the cells, for our purposes, are the cell membranes or walls, the nucleus and the mitochondria. In brief, the membranes surround the total cell and the individual organelles within each cell. The cell membrane is the 'wall' around the whole cell. The mitochondrial membrane is the 'wall' around the mitochondria, and the nuclear membrane is the wall around the nucleus, and so forth.

What do these cell parts do? In summary, this is how the various parts of the cell are arranged.

Working from the outside inwards, we start with the outer cellular membrane, the membrane that surrounds the entire cell. It is the guardian of the cell, it protects the cell from unwanted outside influences. It also allows the passage of substances and information both into and out of the cell, in a controlled way. It allows (a) external compounds needed by the cell into the cell; and (b) cellular compounds that need to be exported, be they metabolic products or waste products, to pass out of the cell. It is also the medium via which each cell communicates with the outside world, via chemical information molecules, and takes information in from the extracellular world, in a similar manner.

Inside this surrounding cellular membrane is the cytoplasm, a general term that covers everything inside the outer cell membrane. It consists of the cytosol and the inner organelles and other structures that lie within it.

The cytosol is the matrix of the cell, in which the nucleus, mitochondria and other organelles are embedded. This used to be called the cytoplasm and be thought of as an amorphous fluid. It is now known to consist of a variety of structural features that hold all the organelles in place, rather like a flexible internal scaffolding, as well as being a fluid medium in which an enormous number of chemical reactions occur, some of which will concern us directly and be discussed later.

The mitochondria will be of particular interest to our story. Most cells, other than red blood cells, have thousands of these. They are where the majority of the oxygen is used and where the majority of the energy of the three food groups, proteins, fats and carbohydrates, is released. They are also the part of the cell that most often fails at the start of the Cancer Process. We will have a lot more to say about these mitochondria later.

The ribosomes will only be mentioned briefly. They are where proteins are built within the cells and many of these proteins, the ones that are enzymes, will be of particular interest to us.

At the core of each cell, again other than red blood cells, is the nucleus. There is only one nucleus to each cell and it contains the genetic material.

Inside each nucleus is a large proportion of your DNA. There is also some DNA in your mitochondria. This mitochondrial DNA is different to the nuclear DNA and we will discuss that later.

Your nuclear DNA is made up of 23 chromosomes.

Each of these chromosomes is made up of several thousand genes.

These genes code for, or are the blueprint for, the formation of the proteins that are made on your ribosomes.

Many of the proteins that these genes code for are enzymes and these play a major role in the way your body functions, in health and in disease and, for our story here, in cancer.

That's it in outline. Now let's consider each of these cellular components in more detail.

The Cell Membrane

Cell membranes are made up of lipids, the proper name for what are commonly referred to as fats. More specifically, the membrane is a bilayer made up of a variety of lipids consisting of triglycerides and their derivatives, known as phosphatides. Triglycerides are made up of three parallel long-chain fatty acids attached at the top rather like a three-pronged fork with the handle removed. The most important derivative is a diglyceride which has only two fatty acids and the third one is replaced by a complex phosphate-rich group. There are four forms of this phosphate-rich group: Phosphatidyl choline, phosphatidyl inositol, phosphatidyl serine and phosphatidyl ethanolamine. I give you these names not because they are an integral part of this story, but because you will see how substances such as choline and inositol, which you may have seen on health food store shelves as supplements, come into the cancer story. It is also pertinent to know the type of fatty acids that form the diglyceride part of the phosphatides. These fatty acids are mainly the essential fatty acids such as linoleic acid and linolenic acid, and other polyunsaturated fatty acids, most commonly found in flaxseed oil. Essential fatty acids, or essential nutrients in general, are ones that you absolutely have to obtain from your diet. You cannot make them yourself, no matter how good the rest of your diet.

These phosphatides line up as a very well organised lipid-lipid bilayer. The free ends of the fatty acids' tails point to the centre and the polar or ionically charged phosphate groups line up on either edge of the bilayer. In between the two layers, rather like the filling in a sandwich, are cholesterol molecules that are integral and essential to the structure of the membrane.

Penetrating into and through the membrane are the communication and transport channels. These channels are made of proteins and make up what are known as receptor sites and receptor channels.

Receptor sites are similar to reception desks in many commercial buildings at which information is received. These protein reception sites respond to messenger molecules passing by in the blood vessels. Messages, in the form of hormones, neurotransmitters and many other somewhat similar compounds, are received here and the information they trigger is passed through the membrane and into the cytoplasm via a sequence of chemical reactions, one sample triggering the next reaction and so on, rather like a domino chain of reactions.

Receptor channels, often also referred to, somewhat confusingly, as receptor sites, are protein tunnels or chains. Compounds can pass and can enter or leave the cells. The receptor channels frequently also act as receptor sites in that they receive or send out information molecules. They can be thought of as messenger receivers ready to pass information through the cell membrane to the inner wall of the membrane. Other messengers inside the cell are then triggered and they take the message further, to other parts of the cell, including the nucleus, as appropriate. This, in a simplified form, is the essence of what happens. In fact the process is enormously complicated, but is a miraculous dance of chemicals performing intricate interlocking sequences of reactions. Be glad of them, they are vital for the healthy functioning of your cells.

Each cell is surrounded by other cells, but also has a blood capillary or blood vessel flowing past part of it. If it was a cube, for instance, one wall would be exposed on the outer side, to the passing bloodstream and the other five sides would be up against neighbouring cells of the same tissue. The part of the cell membrane that is exposed to the passing blood supply is known as the plasma membrane. Cell surface receptors and channels are embedded on, in and through the plasma membrane.

The messenger molecules that bind to receptor sites are known as ligands. Ligands can be peptides (very small proteins), hormones, neurotransmitters, growth factors, cytokines, or a wide variety of other molecules that are either endogenous (internally produced) or exogenous (derived from outside). There are thousands of receptor sites on a single cell's membrane and each is specific for a particular biochemical pathway, reaction or series of reactions within the cell, which they may either activate or block. Receptor channels are selective and monitored.

Once inside the membrane and within the cytoplasm the messenger molecules travel through the cell, usually, but not always, to the nucleus. Here they repeat the process of crossing the membrane, this time the nuclear membrane. Once inside they act on the nucleus, triggering the production of a protein (enzyme) that facilitates the required reaction within the cell.

In summary: the messenger, or ligand, is an external signal, arriving from the bloodstream. Once the external signal is received by a receptor site on the cell membrane it triggers a flow of reactions through the membrane, into the cell's cytosol and so to the nucleus. This process is known as <u>transduction</u>.

As an example, one group of external signalling compounds is made up of compounds called Growth Factors. These are soluble molecules that bind to specific receptor sites (proteins) on the cell's membrane and trigger a sequence of events within the cell. Cell Adhesion Molecules (CAMs) form another group. These are proteins that lie on the cell's surface and control the way that the cell interacts with its environment. They control the amount of contact each cell has with the other cells in the neighbourhood and they inform the cell as to the nature of its surroundings.

Transduction is a normal and healthy process, but in cancer cells the level of signal transduction is often excessive, contributing to the rapid growth and development of cancer cells. The process can be blocked, if required, such as in the inhibition of cancer cells. This can be done by inhibiting the various enzymes involved in transduction, an action that can be accomplished by a number of natural substances, as well as by some medical drugs.

In other words, via the receptors that lie on the surface of, or pass through healthy cell membranes, your cells can learn how to behave appropriately and harmoniously within the total functioning of your body. They obtain information from the outside environment and they communicate with the outside environment. They take in desired compounds and send out important products needed elsewhere. They expel unwanted compounds, waste products of metabolism, and toxins. In general, healthy cells respond appropriately to growth factors from their environment and to CAMs.

This again is a beautifully orchestrated dance of molecules and reaction sequences. It is held within tight control limits by the checks and balances issued by healthy cells. This process also means that your cell membrane is the true master of your cell, the 'brain' behind it, the part of your cell that enables normal healthy cell functioning, up to the maximum of which each of your cells is capable. It also enables the most appropriate interactions and communications between each of your cells and the rest of your body. Healthy cell membranes are vital to health.

Unfortunately, all this can go wrong once cancer starts. Cancer cells can produce their own growth factors and so can dictate their own activity, including growth, reproduction and movement. This also means that they can close themselves off from the information coming from healthy cells, including those of the immune system. Cancer cells are adaptive, as we shall see, and can develop protective strategies. They can, for instance, develop means by which they block the entrance of the drugs and remedies you might use on your road to recovery. Fortunately there are some natural compounds that can counter or reduce this. One of the tests in the Second Test Panel provides information about this, and whether or not you need to block this self-protective reaction of your cancer cells.

From all this it should be clear that healthy cell membranes are a vital part of healthy tissues. A significant part of any recovery protocol should include actions and compounds that contribute to healthy cell membranes. This is one of the reasons why the omega-3 fatty acids in combination with the sulphur amino acids of proteins play such an important role in strengthening the cells against cancer. This combination of foods or nutrients, intimately blended, supplies the membranes with the essential fatty acids in a form that is well absorbed, and in an activated form, required for their optimum function. It can be achieved by blending flaxseed oil with yoghurt, or with a powdered protein such as whey, rice, hemp, or pea protein, mixed in water. This is discussed more fully in the chapter on Dr Budwig in *Cancer Concerns*, the preceding book in this series.

The Mitochondrion

Thus far we have discussed the cell membranes. Now it is time to consider the mitochondrion. There are many other organelles within the cell but the most important organelle type for this chapter, and the discussion of cancer, is the mitochondrion. In a sense, each mitochondrion is a 'captured entity'. It is thought that, way back in our evolutionary history, at the time of single-celled organisms, each mitochondrion had a life of its own as a separate organism. It was an organism that used oxygen for the efficient conversion of organic material into energy. At that time our biological ancestors were not only simple cellular organisms but were anaerobes, functioning without the use of oxygen. They functioned, and derived their energy, from fermentation reactions, instead of oxidative reactions. This was an inefficient form of metabolism and did not allow for much evolutionary advance. In a major evolutionary step forward these anaerobes each engulfed many thousands of mitochondria and made use of them. Specifically they used the mitochondria's very efficient, oxygen-based, energy production reactions to make huge strides in what they could do and how they could evolve.

To this day, energy production in the cytosol, outside the mitochondria, is achieved by anaerobic reactions. But only a limited quantity of energy is produced in this way, possibly around approximately five per cent, not nearly enough for health. Energy produced in the mitochondria is much more efficient and is achieved by oxidative, aerobic reactions. This energy availability is many times that which the cells themselves could achieve via activities in their cytosol.

As a result of their history your mitochondria have their own unique DNA. When sperm and ovum come together in conception the sperm brings with it its nuclear genetic material in the form of DNA, but little else, and certainly no mitochondria. The ovum brings with it its nucleus with its DNA and the mitochondria with their DNA. So your nuclear genes and DNA come from both your father's sperm and your mother's ovum. But all of your mitochondrial DNA is inherited entirely from your mother. For reasons that will now be obvious it is different to the DNA of the nucleus, which you inherited from both your father and your mother.

Virtually all the oxygen taken in by your cells is used and processed by your mitochondria. The rest of each of your cells, including the cytosol and the other organelles within them, are essentially anaerobic, or oxygen-free. Once the early cells had captured their thousands of mitochondria, way back in evolution, they could become supremely efficient oxygen-using organisms. This allowed the huge surge forward in evolution. In our present state the possession of mitochondria is why we need oxygen. The mitochondria are also where more than ninety per cent of the energy from the proteins, fats and carbohydrates that you eat is released and made available. Without mitochondria you would be very sluggish indeed. In cancer it is the mitochondria that become faulty, and this fact compromises the rest of each cell and your overall health.

The three major energy-rich food components are carbohydrates, fats and proteins. The way in which this energy is released in the cells is important in relation to cancer.

Energy production comes from the three major food groups, to a greater or lesser extent. Almost all the complex carbohydrates you absorb are catabolised or broken down within your digestive tract, to produce glucose. Those that are not catabolised in this way, the non-digestible carbohydrates, known colloquially as 'fibre', are not absorbed but travel on to your colon, where they feed the beneficial bacteria and bulk out your stool. Some other carbohydrates, the simple ones such as fructose, agave or corn starch, go to your liver where they are converted into glucose.

The glucose then enters your cells, with the helpful action of insulin and a compound called glucose tolerance factor, via glucose receptor sites or channels and enters the cytosol. This cytosol is anaerobic, that is to say its reactions function in the absence of oxygen. In a chain of reactions commonly known as the Embden-Meyerhof pathway of glycolysis,[4] a 6-carbon glucose molecule is first rearranged, and then partially split into two 3-carbon molecules, called pyruvic acid. At the mitochondrial membrane each of these is then split into a 2-carbon

---

[4] More accurately, but less commonly, referred to as the Embden-Meyerhof-Parnas pathway.

acetyl group with the release of one molecule of carbon dioxide, which in time you will breathe out.

Two compounds are relevant here and will be discussed further in later chapters. When this phase of glucose breakdown occurs incorrectly, your blood level of lactic acid, and of a compound abbreviated to PHI, increases. These are discussed later when we discuss the First Test Panel. The levels of both of these compounds commonly increase in people who either have cancer or are in the early stages of the Cancer Process. They can be used as early warning markers for the disease, as we shall discover.

Citric acid cycle in the mitochondrion

The next phase happens in the mitochondria.

All these acetyl groups enter fully into the mitochondria and then enter the citric acid cycle where they are broken down further. They come from dietary carbohydrates via the above reaction sequence that occurs in the cytosol. They also come from the breakdown of the fatty acids that come from the fats and oils that you eat. One of the most important functions of each mitochondrion is the ultimate breakdown, by oxidation, of these acetyl groups.

The easiest way to picture this cycle is to think of a merry-go-round. Each acetyl group climbs on the first 'horse' and starts round the circle. At different points along the way carbon atoms are released and carried off until, back at the start, they have all gone, and the original 'horse' is empty and ready to receive the next acetyl group.

Dietary proteins are broken down by digestion into individual amino acids. The nitrogen they contain, and the nitrogen from amino acids made in you body, is excreted in your urine. The nature of the remainder of the various amino acid molecules will depend on the nature of the individual amino acid, but one way or another these non-nitrogenous residues all enter the citric acid cycle. In our example, they all clamber onto a horse at some part of the circuit, and are broken down, with the help of oxygen.

The reactions of the citric acid cycle lead to the production of carbon dioxide, by adding oxygen to the carbon in the food carbohydrate, and water, by adding oxygen to the hydrogen in the carbohydrate, and energy.

That is the first part of the mitochondrial breakdown of the various food components. Depending on the nature of your diet, 90% or more of your energy is released from your food in these two phases of mitochondrial function, the citric acid cycle and the electron transport chain discussed below. Less than 10% is released in the cell's cytosol.

Healthy mitochondria are absolutely essential in relation to good health and energy production; they are also essential for the avoidance of cancer.

From this it is clear that once the various food components, the macromolecules of food, the carbohydrates, fats and proteins, have been broken down to smaller components, entered the mitochondria and gone through the citric acid cycle, the end products are essentially the same: water, carbon dioxide and energy.

Most of this energy is released in the form of a large number of high energy molecules called NADPH, NADH and FADH. The energy from only one molecule of glucose leads to the production of a much larger number of these high energy compounds.

The next step, following the production of these three high energy compounds in the citric acid cycle, is to release their energy in smaller and more manageable packages.

The electron transport chain, or the respiratory chain, is the next topic we need to consider. In this sequence of reactions, high energy NADPH releases sufficient energy to convert three molecules of low energy ADP into three molecules of moderate but higher energy ATP. ATP is the general 'energy currency' of your cells and is used to fuel many hundreds, if not thousands, of reactions. NADH also releases sufficient energy to 'recharge' three molecules of low energy ADP up to three molecules of ATP. FADH releases sufficient energy to produce two molecules of ATP from two of ADP.

This electron transport, or respiratory, chain takes place on the inner mitochondrial membrane and is dependent upon its healthy structure and function. So we are back to recognition of the importance of having healthy membranes, both surrounding and within your cells.

It has been suggested by many eminent scientists, starting with Nobel Prize winner Dr Otto Warburg in papers published in the 1930s, that cancer is the result of oxygen deprivation, failure of the respiratory or electron transport chain, at the cellular level, and faulty or inactive mitochondria.

Thus, first detecting, and then correcting, any errors in metabolism within the mitochondria has to be a major focus for both the prevention of, and the recovery from, cancer. This will be discussed later.

These reactions are dependent on cardiolipin, a lipid compound found only in this inner mitochondrial membrane[5] where it constitutes approximately 20 per cent of the lipids present. In a study of brain tumours in mice a significant number of cardiolipin abnormalities were found[1] and these are thought to have contributed to the mitochondrial and respiratory failure that can lead to cancer.

As hinted at above, faulty mitochondria are thought to be an inherent part of the development of cancer. As over ninety per cent of the energy from your food is derived as a result of the processes that occur in the mitochondria, it is no wonder that if you have cancer, with its associated mitochondrial failure, you will, eventually, experience fatigue.

The aerobic production of energy is not the only role of the mitochondria, although it is a major one. They also store calcium. They are important for cell signalling and the synthesis of a number of compounds, such as heme (in haemoglobin) and steroids. Healthy mitochondria are also required for many of the normal actions that

---

[5] Cardiolipin is also found in some bacteria which is relevant in that it is thought that mitochondria may be the descendants of bacteria or bacterial-like organisms that were at an early evolutionary stage incorporated into non-mitochondrial cells. This combination then enabled a major step forward in the evolution of multicellular and more evolved species.

help to prevent cancer, such as apoptosis (the voluntary suicide of cells), to be discussed later.

The Nucleus

The nucleus of each of your cells houses your nuclear genetic material in the form of DNA. DNA is short for deoxyribonucleic acid and it is a double strand or chain of molecules known as nucleotides. These nucleotides in turn are made up of the sugar, deoxyribose, phosphate groups and varying combinations of four bases. The latter, in their various combinations, make up the 'letters' and 'words' of the DNA. Two of these chains are twisted into a spiral or helix and held in place by bonding links between the two chains. RNA, which is short for ribonucleic acid, is, in effect, a single chain, of somewhat similar structure, instead of a double helix. In RNA, deoxyribose is replaced by ribose, and one of the bases is slightly different, but otherwise it is essentially similar to a single strand of DNA.

You may have been thinking, as many people do, that the 'brain' or control centre of your cell is the nucleus, with its DNA. However, this is arguably not so, and it is important to keep this in mind when considering cancer. As discussed above, it can be argued that the membrane of the cell is the real brain of the cell, followed by the membranes of the various organelles within the cell. The nucleus of the cell, often thought of as the 'brain', is in fact the slave of the cell membrane and to a large it extent it obeys the instructions and acts on the information that it receives from this all important membrane.

The main job, though not the only one, of the nucleus is to house the nuclear DNA. This double-stranded helix is made up of 23 chromosome pairs that in turn are, together, made up of approximately 20,000 genes. However, only a few, about 2%, of these genes actually code, or act as blueprints, for proteins. The role of the non-coding genes is still being researched.

Each gene is made up of specific combinations of the four much smaller molecules, the nucleotides. Specific combinations of these four identify or code for individual amino acids, the components of protein molecules. When a protein is being built the string of these four-letter codes is 'read', one after the other, and the appropriate amino acid is added to the growing chain, one after the other. This process continues until the desired protein is built. At which point a specific combination of nucleotides stops the chain formation.

Thus the coding genes on the various chromosomes within the nuclear DNA are essentially passive blueprints for the manufacture of specific proteins. They wait to be activated by outside instructional molecules. A large proportion of these proteins are enzymes that catalyse and thus facilitate specific chemical reactions. Others are structural proteins, such as those of your muscles, skin and organs.

The activity of a gene, known as its expression, is turned on or off by the chemical messengers that arrive from outside the nucleus. The nucleus itself has no on-off switch of its own. It does not act proactively but waits for the instructions that come from elsewhere. These instructions generally come either from some other part of the cell itself, or from an outside messenger molecule via the sequence of reactions that travel through the cell membrane and across the cytosol. The final message stimulates the DNA into activity; a gene is triggered, followed by a sequence of reactions such that the message reaches the ribosomes where the required proteins are to be made.

It is true that if you have a gene that is totally missing, its protein cannot be built, but you would almost certainly know about that from birth. That would be a clear genetic birth defect. If you have a gene that functions poorly or inadequately you may produce insufficient of the required protein, and this we will discuss later. But, overall, the instructions as to how the nucleus will behave come via the cell membranes, and this is an important thought to keep in mind as you read on.

It is worth emphasising this point. The nucleus is where your genes are housed, rather like the data on the hard disk of your computer. Your own brain and fingers operate the keys that tell the hard disk of your computer what to do. Like the hard disk, the nucleus on its own, does nothing, or very little. It is the input from outside the nucleus, the information molecules or ligands, and their impact on each individual cell's membrane and its receptor sites, that tell first the cell and then its nucleus whether to express (activate), or not, the activity of specific genes.

This is how the DNA achieves the desired outcome as it sets off the sequence of events that will create a new protein, needed to encourage a particular reaction. This, in a bit more detail, is how the new protein is made:

Transcription is the first step in this sequence of events. The message comes into the cell, in the form of transcription factors and other epigenetic agents. They act on the cell's membrane and indicate the need for the synthesis of a specific protein or amino acid sequence. For this to be achieved a specific gene has to be activated. This message reaches the nucleus and a specific segment of the DNA double helix chain unzips. This segment forms the template against which the individual nucleotides are brought together and built into a single stranded RNA. In this way messenger RNA, or mRNA, forms. Think of this as being a mould that details the final product in reverse.

Translation is the next step. This mRNA then moves out of the nucleus and travels to a ribosome, the cell organelle where proteins are synthesised, and, rather like a tape fed through the heads of an old-fashioned cassette player, the sequence of groups of four nucleotides along the chain is read and the required amino acids are added on, one after the other until the final protein is produced and then set free. In healthy cells this newly manufactured protein then moves on to where it is required and normal function continues.

When it is time for a cell to divide and produce two daughter cells (they are never called sons), the entire DNA strand has to unzip and each half acts as a template for a copy, in such a way that two molecules of DNA are formed, one for each new daughter cell. They should each be an exact copy of the DNA in the original cell in which they are built.

This is clearly a huge and complex process with many possibilities of error, and in fact many errors do occur, but are corrected. If the procedure does go wrong and is not corrected, faulty or mutated DNA with faulty genes is produced. These faulty genes, in turn, can produce faulty proteins, or may fail to produce certain required proteins, or may produce them in insufficient amounts. This step is critical and is monitored by a compound called protein 53 or p53. We will have more to say about this later, in the information on the

Second Test Panel, but in brief this is what happens: The first action of p53 is to monitor the products of cellular replication. If there is a fault, p53 then triggers reactions that endeavour to repair the problem. If this repair is not successful p53 then triggers a second set of reactions that ensure that the cell destroys itself (apoptosis). If p53 fails to control this DNA replication and faulty cells are allowed to survive, mutations are generally the result and many of these can lead to cancer. A lack of appropriate p53 activity is a common finding in people with cancer.

Genes

The next step in this discussion is to focus on the nature of genes themselves. There is much enthusiasm within the medical profession for the claim that it is your faulty genes that cause cancer and that if therapeutic interventions into the activity of these inherited genes could be accomplished cancer could be prevented. Conversely, there is criticism of this view from other professionals, and you will read more about that later when we consider the two somewhat different theories as to how cancer cells are formed. For now we will consider some of the types and characteristics of some of the relevant genes in relation to cancer.

Cancer cells, once formed, are inherently genetically unstable. This might be thought to make them vulnerable and easy to destroy. However, it also makes them flexible and adaptable so that they can evade or circumvent the activity of chemotherapy agents and related attempts to kill them.

Because their genetic make-up has been altered, they have developed the ability to avoid the normal checks and balances that control healthy cells. This actually increases the likelihood that they will survive and thrive. They will mutate even further whenever they are exposed to a potential mutagen or carcinogen. This characteristic enables them to adapt further to changes, often toxic or harmful ones, in their environment. It means, for instance, that they can develop the ability to avoid the damaging effect of chemotherapeutic agents, radiation or even many natural remedies, thus reducing the effectiveness of these treatments over time. This is one of the challenges that presents itself to those planning recovery programmes.

It is now pertinent to mention, in more detail, the different types of genes, carried on the DNA, both normal and mutated, as they relate to cancer, and to discover what they do.

Genes, as described above, code for the synthesis of specific proteins and these proteins have a variety of functions. Recall that some proteins are essentially structural, such as those involved in the skeleton, the muscles and the various organs through your body including the liver, kidneys and lungs. There are also proteins that are dominantly functional. They are involved in the activity and metabolism of the body. Some of them are messenger molecules, some are hormones, and most, though not all, are biological catalysts or enzymes.

Most of the proteins in which we are interested here are enzymes. Genes can be turned on and off, both in the short and the long term. You may have had some genes all your life that have never been turned on, never functioned. They may remain like that for your entire life. Alternatively, some unusual outside (epigenetic) trigger may cause them to become activated. When turned on they can initiate the production of specific enzyme proteins. When turned off these proteins are not synthesised. If these are genes that facilitate cancer you do not, of course, want to have them turned on.

It may seem strange that we have genes that can facilitate the rapid reproduction and growth of cancer cells, but as you read on you will discover that, in the right time and place, many of them do have a constructive purpose. They offer a benefit, but only when needed and when kept under control.

Enzymes catalyse specific reactions and, as a result, rapidly increase the rate at which these reactions occur. In fact, without them most reactions would occur so slowly that they would not seem to be happening at all and your metabolism could grind to a halt. With them the reactions can occur hundreds of times a second or even more. Thus, when genes are turned on or off the activity of the reactions for which they are responsible is either increased or decreased in a dramatic and profound way. There are genes that code for enzymes that inhibit the development of cancer, and there are those that code for enzymes that facilitate the development of cancerous cells and, ultimately, the growth of a tumour. As you read on you will repeatedly come across oncogenes, proto-oncogenes, tumour suppressor genes and others. In fact we have already touched on them briefly. We will discuss them here in greater detail, specifically as they relate to cancer.

A proto-oncogene is a gene that can turn into a cancer-causing oncogene. Most proto-oncogenes code for proteins that are involved in cell growth and in the differentiation of cells from immature non-specialised cells to mature specialised cells, from adult stem cells to cells of the tissue in which they have been residing and where they are now needed for growth or repair. These proto-oncogenes have an important role to play in healthy cells but their activity is carefully controlled so that the rates of cellular reproduction and tissue growth or repair are kept within the normal required levels. They operate via signal transduction, the process by which a signal or stimulus is converted into another signal or stimulus, usually within the cell and usually catalysed by either a single (protein) enzyme or by a series of enzymes in a signal transduction pathway.

The change from proto-oncogene to oncogene can be triggered by surprisingly small amounts of triggering agents. A single small signal can result in a very larger set of reactions, which can in turn result in an even larger set of reactions by a process known as signal amplification. (Think of the effect of doubling, redoubling and doubling again. The growth rate becomes exponential.)

An oncogene, as its name suggests, is a cancer gene, or, more correctly, a gene that can lead to cancer. It is usually formed from a proto-oncogene, generally either by mutation of the proto-oncogene or by its increased production and increased activity. Either way, an activated oncogene, once formed is capable of encouraging a healthy cell to turn into a cancer cell. An external or epigenetic event is normally required to turn the proto-oncogene into its oncogene form.

The external event is one of the epigenetic factors and is usually an aspect of your overall lifestyle, a harmful aspect that needs correction.

Put more formally, there are three basic ways in which a proto-oncogene can be changed into an oncogene.

- The first is by mutation such that there is a change in the structure or nature of the gene. This in turn creates changes in the protein enzyme that is coded for by the gene. This change may lead to an increase or decrease in the activity of the enzyme, or it may lead to loss of control or regulation of the activity of the enzyme.

- The second is due to an increased concentration of the enzyme, resulting from a lack of control over its synthesis, a process known as misregulation. This misregulation can lead to increased production of the enzyme or to the increased lifespan of the enzyme. This increased concentration of the enzyme can also occur when the gene is duplicated.

- The third way occurs when the chromosome on which the gene occurs is rearranged. As a result, the gene may express itself in the wrong type of cell or under inappropriate circumstances.

There are two aspects of the problem with oncogenes. Firstly, once formed, oncogenes can cause specific damage to cellular chemistry. Secondly, and perhaps more damagingly, once a mutation has been produced, it is common to find that no further input is necessary for the harmful process to continue indefinitely. This is a major matter of concern. The original cell has been mutated and this mutation will be carried on to the daughter cells and beyond, without the input of any further signals, leading to the multiplication of the original transformed (mutated) cell and ongoing tumour growth. This is one of the reasons why simply removing the cause of cancer, the carcinogen, the stress or the faulty lifestyle habit, is rarely sufficient to halt the Cancer Process once it has fully started. Further recovery strategies are required.

Remember also that many activities that are common in embryo development, when rapid cell divisions, multiplication and growth are desirable, can show up in mature but faulty cells that turn into rapidly dividing cancer cells when this same protection of growth characteristics is no longer desirable.

There are, of course, many oncogenes. Mention is made below of a few, some of which we will be discussing or that you can do tests for. If they are found to be present (in mutated form) and at abnormal levels this can lead to indications for the type of positive remedial actions that you may want to incorporate into your recovery plan.

That was the bad news. Now it is time for some good news. There are some helpful genes, known as tumour suppressor genes. These are anti-oncogenes. Their role is to protect the cell from acting in such a way that they become cancer cells. They do this by blocking one of the steps along the pathway that could, if allowed to operate, lead to the formation of cancer cells and the growth of a tumour. The p53 gene is one of the genes tested for in the Second Test Panel, and is one of these suppressor genes. The protein 21 gene is another such suppressor gene.

Examples of tumour suppressor genes:

BAX induces apoptosis by competing with Bcl-2.
It is partially controlled by p53.

Both p53 and BAX are included in the Second Test Panel.

p53 gene codes for p53 which protects and, if needed, initiates the repair of DNA.

It suppresses tumour growth and triggers apoptosis of cells that cannot be repaired. It has the opposite effect when mutated.

Both the wild (normal) and mutated form are part of the Second Test Panel.

p21 gene acts with p53 and can be tested for if required.

However, there is also more bad news. Even these beneficial tumour suppressor genes can be harmed or mutated, in which case their protective effect is lost and the cell can then turn into a cancer cell. This mutation does not generally occur on its own. It can do so under the action of a cancer-causing agent, a carcinogen or related toxin, or a sequence of damaging reactions that is no longer blocked by the activity of the tumour-suppressing anti-oncogene. That is why, in the Second Test Panel, the mutated form of p53 is tested for, as well as the wild or normal form.

Oncogenes in more detail:

Bcl-2 inhibits apoptosis, protects cancer cells from free radical damage.

It is partially controlled by p53.

Both p53 and Bcl-2 are included in the Second Test Panel.

fos and *jun*	These enzymes are briefly stimulated by growth factors. The proteins are transcription factors and encourage the start of the cell cycle and proliferation.
	In excess they lead to uncontrolled proliferation. They are transient.
HER-2/neu	common in about a third of breast tumours.
	It stimulates transduction and is associated with a poor prognosis.
MDM2	binds to, inhibits and destroys p53. When the protective action of p53 is needed the binding of MDM2 to p53 is blocked, the level of p53 rises and apoptosis is stimulated. This gene is over-expressed in cancer thus reducing the beneficial action of p53.
Myc or c-myc	affects cell proliferation, differentiation, and apoptosis. It is needed to initiate cell division and to prevent differentiation.

A transcription factor. It binds to DNA and so controls the flow of genetic information from DNA to mRNA.

The mutated oncogene form leads to loss of regulation of many other genes including some whose dysregulation leads to cancer.

The mutated from of Myc is found in many tumours as the oncogene form leads to increased DNA synthesis and abnormal chromosomes.

It may stimulate the production of collagenases and thus stimulate metastatic invasion, increase the expression of MDM2 genes and inhibit apoptosis.

WNT   WNT proteins are involved in cancer and in embryo development as well as in some normal adult processes.

Mutations

A number of genetic errors can lead to excessive cell proliferation and the development of cancer. Some have already been referred to, but it is helpful to group them together here, particularly as they are components of the test panels to be described later.

One of these mutations concerns p53. Recall that protein 53 is a major protective protein. It resides in the nucleus and monitors the replication of DNA and the formation of daughter cells. If or when a fault is detected in the DNA replication, p53 has two options. Firstly it tries to correct the fault. If this is unsuccessful it then triggers apoptosis, the destruction of the faulty cell. A major error occurs either when the level of p53 production is inadequate, or when the p53 gene is mutated. As a result of either of these situations faulty cells are not detected, or, if they are, they are neither corrected nor destroyed; instead they are allowed to live on and multiply.

The second example concerns BAX and Bcl-2 genes. The BAX protein, coded for by the BAX gene, stimulates apoptosis and helps to prevent the replication or build up of faulty cells. Bcl-2 protein acts against BAX and inhibits apoptosis. When reduced production of BAX or excessive production of Bcl-2 occurs there is reduced cell suicide or apoptosis and faulty cells are able to thrive and reproduce.

Thirdly, genetic errors can lead to increased production of proteins that stimulate angiogenesis, such as vascular endothelial growth factor (VEGF). When this happens there is increased angiogenesis leading to a generous supply of new blood to fuel and nourish the growing tumour.

The Second Test Panel includes tests for the levels of the BAX, Bcl-2 and VEGF genes.

Transcription factors act as switches within the cell's nucleus that turn the expression of specific genes on or off. In cancer cells, they commonly stimulate the expression of oncogenes and inhibit the expression of tumour suppressor genes, both of which actions are harmful.

Methylation

There is another way that the activity of genes can be controlled, at least in the long term. When methyl groups are added to the relevant section of DNA a gene can become less active. When the methyl groups are removed gene expression is increased. In general, oncogenes tend to be under-methylated and so are over active. Transforming growth factor beta (TGF-beta), for example, a gene that reduces cell proliferation, can be over-methylated and so become underactive and fail to halt excessive cellular proliferation.[2]

We started this section by talking about the genetic instability of cancer cells. The maintenance of healthy tissues depends on the reduction of this pro-cancerous genetic instability. One way to achieve this is to reduce oxidative stress. This is caused by the action of oxidising agents and the production, presence and activity of free radicals. This is partly why there is such an emphasis, in CAM therapies, on anti-oxidants in the promotion of health. The more oxidising of the environment, the greater the genetic instability and the greater the risk of mutations forming. The more anti-oxidants, derived mainly from vegetables and fruits in the diet, the greater is the chance of increasing genetic stability and of avoiding mutations.

Before leaving this section it is important to make one more point. An excessively oxidising environment can be dangerous. However, your cells do need oxygen, your mitochondria need it and without it they fail to function and your cells can turn to anaerobic activity and cancer. The answer to this seeming conflict is to have sufficient anti-oxidants in your diet to protect your healthy tissues from the adverse effects of unwanted oxidising reactions, while at the same time contributing to the smooth functioning of your mitochondria and their efficient utilisation of oxygen for the production of energy.

That was a discussion of the cells in your body and some of their internal components. We will now consider genes in relation to cancer more closely and from a more practical perspective and bring some of these ideas together.

CHAPTER 4

CANCER DEVELOPMENT

You now know something about your cells, about their structure and the way that they function. You also know something about the structure of your genes and the way that they too function. You know at least enough to be able to develop a deeper understanding of cancer and the way you can deal with it.

Cancer is Unique

Cancer is unique among health problems. Almost any other health problem is a problem *of* an organ or tissue. Cancer is a health problem that develops *on* or *at* an organ or tissue, grows on that tissue and damages that tissue. It is not primarily a failure of function of a particular tissue or organ. What does this mean?

If you have Type-I diabetes there is primarily a problem with your pancreas and the way it functions relating to the amount or type of insulin it produces. The treatment focuses on improving the function of your pancreas and its insulin production. If you have heart disease it is a problem of the way your heart and arteries function and the treatment aim is to improve the state of your arteries and improve cardiac function. If you have a thyroid problem then the treatment focus is on improving its response to thyroid-stimulating hormone and its output of the thyroid hormones. The same is true of diseases of the kidneys, liver or other organs. If you have arthritis the treatment aim is to improve the function and structure of the arthritic joints. If you have asthma the treatment is focused on improving lung health and function.

Cancer is different. If you have breast cancer it is not because your breasts are failing in their job and you do not focus on improving the function of your breasts and their production of milk. It is because a tumour has grown in or on your breast. If you have lung cancer you do not focus on improving lung function, at least as a primary treatment option. You do not have prostate cancer because your prostate function is compromised and your treatment does not focus on improving prostate function. If you have colon cancer you are not given treatments that are primarily focused on increasing the level of fibre in your diet and the frequency of your stool.

Cancer is not the result of the failure of the organ or tissue where the tumour is located. The tumour comes first. The local tissue may then become damaged and its function may become compromised. If you have breast cancer and a young baby, your milk production may become problematic as a result of the cancer. If you have lung cancer your lung function, your breathing and your intake of oxygen may become compromised, but the tumour came first, function was reduced as a result of the cancer. If you have prostate cancer the tumour may interfere with the function of your prostate, but this is a result of the cancer, not the cause of the cancer. If a tumour grows in your colon it may well compromise or damage your colon and its ability to function, but again the tumour came first, then the failure in function.

In other words, you may, as the cancer progresses, have problems with the way the various organs or tissues function, but that is because the cancer has lodged or grown in that location and *then* compromised the function of that tissue. If a tumour grows in your breast it may become misshapen. If you have tumours in your lungs they may cease to function correctly. Similarly, your colon or prostate may not function correctly *because* cancer has developed there.

This is an important point to make, and it is valid, even if you argue that a clogged up colon can contribute to cancer. This is true, but it can contribute to cancer *anywhere in the body*, not necessarily where the blockage is most common. If your liver function is inadequate, and it fails to remove toxins from your body, this may contribute to cancer anywhere in the body, not necessarily in the liver.

This shows up an important aspect of cancer. It is a systemic disease, at least initially. Cancer is not a localised disease, at least not at the start. Granted, it may show up, in time, as a tumour at a specific location, but it starts out as a cellular disease and these cellular changes can occur in almost any or all types of cell throughout the body. This concept is of fundamental importance, and leads on, as you will learn later, to the way we can test for the earliest signs of cancer by using blood and urine tests that provide information about the whole body via the activity of the cells in general.

Cancer as a Process

There are, in general, two types of tumour: benign tumours and malignant tumours. A distinction is made between them. A benign tumour is not as harmless as it sounds, it can do local, space-occupying, damage, but it is enclosed and not likely to spread or metastasise. A malignant tumour is one that is capable of metastasising, of spreading throughout your body, and so of doing life-threatening damage. This further highlights the fact that the problem of cancer is the effect of the cancerous cells on the tissue, to which it travels, or on or at which tissue it is located, not, primarily, a problem of that organ or tissue itself.

Setting aside the less common cancers, such as those of the blood and lymphatic system, in most people's minds having cancer involves having a tumour. In the medical approach cancer is diagnosed by the presence of a malignant tumour. The detection focus is on finding a tumour. The aim of the medical approach to treatment is focused on eradicating the tumour, on removing or destroying it. Relatively little thought is given as to how or why you developed the tumour, or the process by which the tumour formed. And it is rare that any of these concepts are taken into account when you or your medical team are planning either recovery or the prevention of a recurrence.

It is the contention of this thesis, and expressed in the previous two books in this series, that it is more useful and more accurate to consider cancer to be a process. This was mentioned in the introductory overview (Chapter One). It is now time to explore this concept further.

There are two phases to this Cancer Process.

In Phase I you do not have cancer, but your state of health, at the cellular level, is such that you are heading towards it, and that any further damaging factors could stimulate the production of active cancer cells more readily than if you were totally healthy, again at the cellular level.

Contributing factors to Phase I are Risk Factors and Predisposing Factors. To some extent there is overlap between the two, but it is still worth considering them both separately.

<u>Risk Factors</u>

Risk Factors are frequently discussed and well documented in the general press and an already established part of the concerns in regard to the development of cancer. They include many historical aspects of your life and, to a larger extent than is true of Predisposing Factors, they are things over which you had limited control. They include such things as your age, sex, a family history of cancer, whether or not a woman had children or breastfed them, a history of infectious agents such as HIV, HPV or *Helicobacter pylori*, a previous high level of radiation exposure, the use of toxic chemicals either in the workplace or round the land or the home, and the use of tobacco. Risk Factors are generally accepted, by individuals and by the medical and other health professions, as having the potential to contribute to cancer. Some of them might not have been operative or present in your life, had you acted differently in the past, others you could not have controlled. They remain in the past and, in most instances, there is little you can do about them now. You can give up tobacco, you can avoid some of the known carcinogens, but you cannot change your age, sex or your history of childbearing and rearing. Nor can you undo your past exposure to damaging radiation or carcinogens.

Many of the Risk Factors are known carcinogens. Ironically they include chemotherapy and radiation therapy, both of which are known to cause cancer. These two treatments might seem to reduce the size of an existing tumour, even to the point where it is too small to be detected, but then be shown, months or years later, to have contributed to or triggered a repeat of cancer.

A family history of cancer is included in the list of Risk Factors, but this need not necessarily be genetic, and this merits comment in the light of the above discussion on genes. Such a history or association could just as well be due to other shared factors, such as the inherited lifestyle, or inherited vulnerability to some of the Predisposing Factors (see below) and the way stress is handled. The solution is to resolve these Predisposing Factors.

To avoid cancer it is helpful if you become conversant with all the Risk Factors that might still apply to you and do all you can to avoid or eliminate them from your lifestyle.

Predisposing Factors

The concept of Predisposing Factors, as an identified group, is newer. The more we learn about cancer the more we learn about the dangers of these Predisposing Factors. They are discussed in detail in *Vital Signs for Cancer*. A brief description is given here. Predisposing Factors do not necessarily lead to cancer, but they may. They may also lead to a number of other degenerative diseases. They certainly do lead to less than optimal health and they leave you vulnerable to picking up infections or to succumbing to other triggers, some of which do stimulate cancer. They leave your body in a state where it has reduced capacity to deal with any other challenges and an increased likelihood of developing cancer and other degenerative diseases.

Predisposing Factors include the following:

Poor diet:

There are many possible errors of diet. Glucose feeds cancer. Therefore a high intake of sucrose (table sugar) or other refined carbohydrates, which provide a sudden rise in blood glucose level, is a serious Predisposing Factor. It is particularly harmful if you already have cancer, even if it is unsuspected and not yet diagnosed. Almost everyone I speak with eats more sugar than they realise as so much is hidden in the foods of commerce. It occurs in unlikely foods. It also masquerades under a number of names, designed to lull you into a false sense of safety. Such names include dextrose, dextrins, maltose, fructose, agave, evaporated cane juice, corn syrup and more. If you manage to avoid these sugars you may still be consuming more sugar than you realise. You may be eating so-called 'health bars' with a high content of dried fruits that have relatively little nutrient value but a high sugar content.

Many fats are bad, particularly those that have been processed, hydrogenated or over-heated. The best ones to use are flaxseed oil, coconut oil, olive oil or butter (organic). Flaxseed oil should be kept in the deep freeze once a bottle has been opened. It melts well below 0°C, and so melts very quickly when exposed to room temperature or if the bottle is put in a bowl of cold water for a few minutes, so it is easy to use. Avoid crisps, chips, fried foods, and most animal fats that have been exposed to a high temperature. There is much more that could be said about a poor diet, but space does not permit, and many other books have been written on this.

Nutrient deficiencies:

Nutrient deficiencies include deficiencies of vitamins and minerals, many of which are needed for the healthy function of the cells in general and, in particular, healthy mitochondria. They will be discussed further, later in this book. Such nutrients also include many of the beneficial compounds, generally referred to as phytonutrients, found in food, particularly in vegetables, herbs and fruit. They are not defined as 'essential for life', meaning that, if everything else in your life was perfect you would probably not die for lack of these. Hence they are not considered to be essential nutrients in the strict sense of the word. Yet hundreds of these phytonutrients are known to provide significant health benefits and help to protect you from other deficiencies or the intake of harmful substances. One example will suffice. The French chemist, Masquelier[3], found that when a diet rich in pycnogenols (some of these phytonutrients, found in such foods as grape seeds and skin and many other sources of vitamin C) were added to vitamin C, the vitamin C was eleven times more effective. This also points to the value of choosing, whenever possible, supplements derived from whole food sources such that they contain all the possible phytonutrients, both known and unknown.

Poor digestion:

Poor digestion has the potential to exacerbate nutrient deficiencies. It may lead to a failure to break down the foods satisfactorily and so fail to release their nutrients. Or it may simply interfere with the absorption of these nutrients.

Poor digestion is also the indicator of other problems. There may be toxins in the digestive tract, including *Candida albicans* and other moulds that can cause harm. You may lack sufficient numbers of the beneficial bacteria that not only keep your gut healthy and aid in the process of digestion but also supply you with nutrients including many of the B group vitamins, and particularly biotin, of which you acquire relatively little from your food. Poor digestion can lead to constipation, with its inherent problems, and to other Predisposing Factors such as IBS.

Poor liver function:

Your liver has more jobs to do than any other organ in your body. See my book *Liver Detox Plan*, in which I discussed this in detail. Your liver is involved in the digestion and absorption of many food components, in the processing of fats, sugars and the amino acids of protein. It stores many of the trace nutrients such as the B group vitamins (hence good quality liver is a nutrient-dense food) and a number of trace minerals. It synthesises a number of protein carriers that are needed to transport nutrients, such as zinc, round your body. It is an active participant in immune function, hormone function; it is an important part of your ability to downgrade and eliminate a variety of toxins, and more, much more. A healthy liver can help to protect you from a wide range of health problems, so look after it if you want to avoid cancer.

The presence of toxins:

Many toxins are known carcinogens. Many more are as yet unrecognised carcinogens. For instance, when I was a geochemist involved in mineral exploration and the analysis of thousands of soil, stream and plant samples for trace levels of many different minerals we did thousands of analyses using carbon tetrachloride as a solvent. As far as we knew then, apart from the rather unpleasant smell, this presented no problem. It is now recognised as a carcinogen and handled much more carefully. The same can be said of many other chemicals. Many chemicals have been put into the marketplace, whether for industrial, agricultural or home use, and only years later found to be much more harmful than was expected.

The toxins to which you may have been exposed, or are still being exposed, include such chemicals, found in the atmosphere, the workplace, marketplace and the home. The term also covers micro-organisms, viruses, bacteria, moulds, worms and other parasites to name a few.

Poor glucose metabolism:

Glucose feeds cancer. Cancer cells derive virtually all their energy from glucose. To facilitate their demand for glucose not only do they have many more receptor sites for glucose than do healthy cells, they also produce their own insulin to increase their glucose uptake further. This is one of the reasons why a low carbohydrate diet, especially one low in refined carbohydrates such as all the different sugars, and grain products such as white flour, white rice and white pasta, is beneficial. A ketogenic diet, based on moderate amounts of good quality protein, be it plant protein or fish and selected meats, combined with very generous amounts of vegetables, herbs and fruits, is to be encouraged.

Stress and adrenal exhaustion:

Dr Fryda (see *Cancer Concerns*) postulated that stress, leading to adrenal exhaustion, is a leading cause of cancer. It causes hormone changes and upsets the balance between adrenalin and noradrenalin. As a result, and in ways that are explained in *Cancer Concerns*, cells became deprived of oxygen and have to develop in such a way that they can store glucose. They do this by converting it to glycogen. Without oxygen they catabolise glucose very inefficiently and obtain only a small amount of its energy. In the process they produce lactic acid which in turn leads to increased mitosis (the development of new daughter cells). This gives them more cells in which to store the glycogen but also leads to the production of even more lactic acid and hence increasingly rapid tissue or tumour growth.

An underactive thyroid gland:

Many people suffer from an unrecognised suboptimal thyroid function. This is partly due to a low intake of the nutrients needed by the thyroid gland such as iodine, copper and zinc, and to other of the Predisposing Factors listed above. It is also due to a failure of diagnosis as the medical parameters for what is taken to be the range of normal levels of the active compounds is too wide. An excellent book, written many years ago, by Dr Broda Barnes[4] discussed this in detail. Ironically, there are simple plant remedies that can boost thyroid function back up to normal, but because the problem is not properly recognised or diagnosed, very few people seek such a remedy.

Poor immune function:

Many people assume that cancer is the result of a failure of immune function. In part this is true. However, cancer cells have managed to develop a number of strategies to avoid detection by the immune system and so to escape destruction. Nonetheless, a healthy immune system has a powerful role to play in preventing cancer, or recovering from it. Thus poor immune function is definitely a Predisposing Factor.

Emotional issues:

It can be argued that there is no health problem that is not associated with some emotional issues. Any form of stress or unhappy thought immediately alters the flow of hormones, the activity of white blood cells and the function of your immune system in general, and initiates other cellular changes. Many of the alternative approaches to cancer recovery will focus on dealing with such emotional issues as an essential part of the strategy. This interaction was discussed in detail in my books *From Stress to Success* and *Choosing Health Intentionally*.

It is possible to consider other Predisposing Factors, but this short outline covers the majority of the main ones. Again, see my book *Vital Signs for Cancer* for a much more detailed description of each of them. In that book you will also find indications for testing which of them might apply to you.

If you recognise these Predisposing Factors in yourself, now is the time to make corrections. It is much easier to do this at this stage than once fully cancerous cells have formed.

Phase Two of the Cancer Process starts at the start of the first faulty cell that is not destroyed but allowed to flourish. It continues to the creation and growth of a detectable and metastatic tumour.

Note that both the Risk Factors and the Predisposing Factors are external aspects of your lifestyle over which you can have a significant, if not total, control, if you choose to act in ways that are beneficial to your health, and remember that many practitioners believe that well over 90 per cent of all cancers are caused by such epigenetic factors.

CHAPTER 5

HOW CANCER STARTS

There are, essentially, only two main types of cells that can turn into cancer cells. These are immature, undifferentiated (as-yet unspecialised) stem cells and mature, differentiated (specialised) cells that have dedifferentiated. Both these cells types occur throughout your body in almost all tissues.

Stem Cells

Stem cells are undifferentiated, non-specialised cells. Think of them as being held in reserve, back-up forces or cells that can be turned (differentiated or specialised) into any new cells that are required. There are three possible ways in which they can divide and multiply.

1. They can divide asymmetrically in such a way that one of the two daughter cells is another stem cell, a copy of themselves, and the other daughter cell is a cell that can develop into a cell of the tissue that is required, such as for wound healing or growth.
2. They can divide symmetrically to produce two daughter cells that can differentiate into the required tissue. However, this would eventually deplete the store of reserve or back-up stem cells. So fortunately there is a third option.
3. They can divide symmetrically in such a way that they produce two daughter stem cells, identical to themselves and so make up the numbers by option (2) above.

Put simply, there are two types of stem cells.

1. <u>Embryonic stem cells</u> are found in the blastocysts which are formed from day five of embryo development and consist of approximately 70 to 100 cells. They are pluripotent, meaning that they can specialise into almost all tissue types. These stem cells can be extracted from the umbilical cord at or just after birth.
2. <u>Mature or adult stem cells</u> are the silent, back-up stem cells referred to above. They are found, quiescent and undifferentiated,

throughout the body tissues. Progenitor cells, developed from adult stem cells, are already partially differentiated. Whereas stem cells can divide and multiply indefinitely, progenitor cells have already lost this ability and can only multiply a finite number of times.

Stem cells and progenitor cells are available to the tissues whenever repair or renewal of specialised cells is required.

Totipotent stem cells are cells that are capable of subdividing and differentiating to produce all the different cell types throughout the body. They are produced by the combining of an ovum and a sperm cell. They can differentiate into both embryonic stem cells and extra-embryonic stem cells and are capable of building up into a total organism.[5]

Pluripotent stem cells have developed from totipotent stem cells and can differentiate into nearly, but not all, cell types.

Multipotent stem cells are somewhat more specialised than pluripotent stem cells and can only specialise or differentiate into cells that are of a somewhat similar type.

Oligopotent stem cells can differentiate into only a very few cell types.

Unipotent stem cells can only produce more of their own cell type, but they still retain some renewal characteristics of stem cells.

Because stem cells are the undifferentiated or partially differentiated cells that are waiting in the wings, they do not yet have the characteristics of any particular tissue. They are not lung, liver, muscle or glandular cells. Like newborn babies, they have not yet specialised in any particular form or skill. Their life path and potential, their chosen career and characteristics are as yet undecided. Cellular decisions as to the way in which they will develop are still ahead of them.

Since stem cells are undifferentiated cells with the ability to turn into almost any type of cell with their lack of specialisation they are ready, when required, to turn into fully operative differentiated or specialised cells. They can turn into the cells of the local tissue when new replacement cells are needed. Stem cells can multiply as required. As this process of specialisation or differentiation progresses they gradually show more and more of the characteristics of the host tissue cell type of which they are to become a part. As this specialisation increases they lose, progressively, the ability to divide and produce daughter cells. This is an important characteristic. Fully differentiated cells of a specific tissue rarely reproduce themselves. The local stem cells are there to provide new cells when these are needed. This is important when we consider cancer.

It is common to find that cancer cells in the breast have at least some of the characteristics of breast cells. However, it is now recognised that these cells were not necessarily, at one time, fully differentiated breast cells that had become less differentiated and turned into cancer cells. It is now recognised that they could also have been stem cells that started to develop into breast cells but became faulty along the way. Similarly, at a metastatic location it may be that the cells show some of the characteristics of the original tumour from the source tissue or location, but that these are the characteristics of the partially differentiated stem cells as well as the dedifferentiated cells of the original tissue.

How a Healthy Cell Becomes a Cancer Cell

The next question relates to how and why:

(a) a healthy stem cell should differentiate in such a way that it incorporates errors and turns into a cancer cell; and

(b) why a healthy mature cell should dedifferentiate, and develop faults, to a point where it can become a potential cancer cell and can then reproduce itself in ways that have the characteristics and capabilities of a cancer cell.

The cause of either of these actions can lie either inside or outside your body. By 'inside', is usually meant inside your cells and specifically inside the nucleus and on your gene, thus 'genetic factors'. By 'outside' is usually meant factors external to your body, thus 'epigenetic factors' and they include all aspects of your lifestyle and diet. Genetic or epigenetic: inside your body and part of your inherited genome or outside your body and part of your lifestyle and emotional make-up, part of the Risk Factors and Predisposing Factors discussed above. There is really no other possibility.

<u>Genes or epigenetics</u>

If you assume that cancer is entirely a genetic inherited trait there is little you can do. If the cause is partly genetic, that is to say if your genes predispose you to cancer but do not mean you will absolutely certainly get cancer, and partly due to epigenetic factors, then you can certainly work on the latter. If cancer is caused entirely by epigenetic factors and has little to do with your genes you can have a major impact on your health and the avoidance of cancer and recovery from it.

The medical profession focuses largely on genetic problems in relation to cancer. However, it is totally possible and highly likely that cancer is largely due to epigenetic factors. In fact, many studies and statistical analyses put this figure well above 60% and some put it as high as 93%.

There are indeed some cancers that are made more likely by the presence of certain genes. However, even with these, and if the genetic make-up increases the likelihood of cancer, cases are known where an individual with such genes has not developed cancer. Thus it is likely that epigenetic factors also play a role. An example of this, and one of the best known, involves the genes that code for breast cancer type 1 and breast cancer type 2 susceptibility proteins, known as BRCA1 and BRCA2. These are both important proteins in protecting you from the development of cancer, and so the genes that code for them are also important. The BRCA1 is a caretaker gene. It codes for the synthesis of a protein, called 'breast cancer type 1 susceptibility protein'. This protein plays a role either in the repair of any damaged or faulty DNA, or the destruction of the faulty cell. BRCA2 is a tumour suppressor gene that has an important role to play in the repair of chromosomal and DNA damage. If either of these genes is mutated, and several hundred different types of mutations have been identified, it increases the individual's risk of developing several types of cancer.

Yet even here, it is unlikely that genes tell the full story. One study showed that 73% of patients who were carriers of the mutated gene had a moderate or strong family history of breast cancer, 28% had little or no family history of cancer, leading to the suggestion of possible modifying genes or contributory environmental facts. In another study, comparison of age of onset for mother/daughter pairs show a decreasing age of onset among the daughters of each pair, leading these authors to suggest possible contributing environmental or epigenetic factors[6] such as could have occurred at a younger age, due to adverse changes in lifestyle and diet.

Overall there is little convincing evidence that your genes are the ultimate cause of cancer. What we will find is that cellular changes, due to epigenetic errors, change your cellular chemistry in such a way that valuable and protective genes are mutated or damaged, proto-oncogenes are stimulated and turned into oncogenes or that otherwise quiescent oncogenes are stimulated into activity.

So let us consider how cancer could develop without the causative factor being faulty genes.

Dr Otto Warburg's Theory, and Beyond

Recall that inside each cell there are many different organelles, just as people have different organs within their body. One type of cell organelle is the mitochondrion. Most of the cell's functions occur without the need for oxygen, yet you know that you need to breathe in oxygen to survive. It is the mitochondria that need this oxygen. Oxygen is vital for their function.

Recall also that glucose is the ultimate end product of the digestion of all forms of sugars, including sucrose or table sugar, dextrose, fructose, laevulose, agave, lactose, galactose, maltose and dextrins. It is also the ultimate product of the digestion of starches, such as those derived from grains, flour, rice, pasta and so forth and from starchy vegetables and fruits such as potatoes, parsnips and bananas.

Of the commonly available food sugars, xylitol, coming into prominence as a 'safe sugar', needs comment. It is actually a sugar alcohol, as its name implies (ending in -ol instead of -ose as do the sugars). It is a five-carbon compound, as opposed to the six-carbon sugars, and only by very indirect and commonly relatively inactive mechanisms can it be converted into the dangerous glucose that feeds cancer cells.

For our present purposes here we need to think back to Chapter Three when we discussed the mitochondrion and reconsider just how your cells handle this glucose.

You will recall that a small amount of glucose breakdown, and a release of a minor amount of the energy it contains, occurs in the anaerobic cytosol. The majority of the energy you derive from your food occurs in the aerobic mitochondria, via first the citric acid cycle and then the electron transport chain.

It is important, for good health, that these reaction sequences occur correctly and that the process is completed without errors.

Nobel Prize winner Dr Otto Warburg, as far back as the 1920s, believed that the ultimate cause of cancer resided in the mitochondria. He stated that cancer was due to a failure of the electron transport chain and the resulting failure of mitochondrial function.[7]

Healthy cells, with a healthy electron transport chain and healthy mitochondria, absolutely need oxygen to function correctly. Cancer cells can live without oxygen and can thrive in a low-oxygen environment, even without any oxygen. In fact, this is a critical distinction between healthy cells and cancer cells.

Cancer cells can derive a major proportion of their energy in the cytosol, within the cell but outside the mitochondria. Healthy cells derive almost all of their energy, as ATP, from the aerobic citric acid cycle inside the oxygen-rich mitochondria, via oxidative phosphorylation and the electron transport chain.

Warburg postulated that the lack of oxygen caused healthy cells to revert to an increased dependency on glycolysis and the cytosol's

Embden-Meyerhof (E-M) pathway for energy production and thus become cancer cells.[8] He stated that, "...*the cause of cancer is no longer a mystery, we know it occurs whenever any cell is denied 60% of its oxygen requirements*"[9], and "*Cancer, above all other diseases, has countless secondary causes. But, even for cancer, there is only one prime cause. ...the prime cause of cancer is the replacement of the respiration of oxygen in normal body cells by a fermentation of sugar* [glucose]."[10]

Every time Dr Warburg put healthy cells in a controlled laboratory environment and totally deprived them of oxygen he found that they had turned into cancer cells. They reverted back to being undifferentiated cells, eminently capable of repeated uncontrolled replications and multiplying to form a tumour. With an adequate supply of oxygen they reverted back to aerobically functioning healthy cells. Modern research continues to prove Warburg's theory.[11]

An alternative theory is that it is fundamentally mitochondrial damage, rather than oxygen deprivation, that leads to cancer.[12] This is rather like the debate as to whether the chicken or the egg came first, the two are inextricably linked. However, it is known that if mitochondria are deprived of oxygen for any extended period of time they suffer irreversible damage.[13]

Gatenby and Gillies have pointed out that increased glycolysis and increased activity of the cytosol's E-M pathway is a common feature of both primary and metastatic cancer cells, and that this is one of the reasons that cancer cells are so glucose hungry. They suggest that this is a means by which pre-malignant cells can adapt to an inadequate supply of oxygen, even intermittently. This increased glycolysis leads to local (lactic) acidosis and the cells then, due to this lactic acid, have increased capacity to multiply and to invade.[14]

Seyfried carried these ideas forward in 2010 and provided further evidence for mitochondrial failure and impaired electron transport chain, with the resulting disordered energy metabolism, as the ultimate cause of cancer. An in-depth, academic and thoroughly referenced discussion of this topic can be found in his book *Cancer as a Metabolic Disease*.[15]

This topic is discussed and referenced in further detail in Section II of this book under 'The Warburg Effect'.

Warburg postulated that there were several reasons behind these failures:

* Oxygen deficiency at the cellular level.
* Deficiency of the nutrients needed for mitochondrial function, what Warburg called the 'essential factors'. Vitamins were only just being discovered in the 1930s and were probably not named in the late 1920s when he was proposing his theory. However, it was obviously known that certain essential factors were needed for correct mitochondrial function.

These essential nutrients include at the most immediate level of involvement: vitamins B1, B2, B3, B5, biotin, CoQ-10, lipoic acid and a number of trace elements. Other nutrient deficiencies can have a more indirect impact.

* A wide variety of toxins.
* Emotional issues.

Ninety years later his ideas are still totally relevant.

One might ask, if this is so, why it is not more widely recognised. For part of the answer, read the story in Section II of two French professors, Pasteur and Béchamp. In the mid-nineteenth century they proposed two alternative theories as to the origin of disease. In brief, Pasteur's theory put micro-organisms as the cause. Béchamp's theory put the poor health and nourishment of the individual as the cause and stated that the micro-organisms were simply making the most of this diseased or weakened state. Later, Pasteur came to acknowledge that he thought Béchamp's theory was the right one. However, the medical and drug companies saw an opportunity if they embraced Pasteur's ideas. They could make and patent drugs that would kill the micro-organisms. They saw no benefit if they embraced Béchamp's theory. You cannot patent or profit from advocating lifestyle improvements. So the drug companies embraced the former. They still do so today even though this is more costly for healthcare providers, places little or no emphasis on prevention and the building of overall good health, and leads to a number of toxic effects, many of them fatal, from the drugs that are administered.

Similarly, an approach to cancer that involves ensuring sufficient cellular oxygen, the supply of essential (non-patentable) nutrients and the elimination of toxins can lead to little or no profit for surgeons, the drug companies that produce the chemotherapeutic agents or the suppliers of radiation equipment and treatments. The view that there is little or nothing that the individual can do to prevent or recover from cancer, and that they should rely on chemotherapy and radiation is enormously profitable for those supplying the common treatments.

Furthermore, the assumption that cancer is caused by faulty genes can lead to funding for enormous amounts of research into gene chemistry, much of it having little or nothing to do, in the long term, with the cause or successful treatment of cancer.

That covers the initial cause of cancer. It is mitochondrial damage, not your inherited genes. However, at the second stage your genes do come into play. There are many consequences of this mitochondrial damage and a large number of them lead to the genetic changes that the medical profession frequently focuses on as the primary, rather than the secondary, cause of cancer. These genetic changes may indeed be involved in cancer, but, it is worth repeating, they are not the prime cause but the consequence of the epigenetic factors and mitochondrial failures as was described by Dr Otto Warburg in the late 1920s and early 1930s.

Let's now take a look at this in more detail. Understanding and utilising these concepts gives us two useful tools. It provides a foundation on which to build the tests that constitute the early warning signs for cancer. It also gives us indications as to the most appropriate CAM therapeutic interventions. These topics will be discussed later.

The development of viable cancer cells is assisted by:

1. A low-oxygen, anaerobic environment

Having sufficient oxygen does not simply mean taking lots of deep breaths, although habitual deep breathing does, of course, help. Aerobic exercise helps, so does yoga breathing. Most people take in only very shallow breaths, and then let them out again rapidly, using only the top ten to twenty per cent of their lungs. Practice taking deep breaths, holding them for longer than you usually do. Then let them out, and immediately breathe in again. This provides the longest amount of time with the air in your lungs. The oxygen in it can then cross the walls of the tiny blood vessels in your alveoli. You cannot absorb oxygen while your lungs are empty, as they probably are for a great proportion of the time in your normal breathing pattern.

2. A lack of essential nutrients:

a) Impaired electron transport chain (the mitochondrial respiratory chain)

The electron transport chain requires a number of nutrients for its function. It can be compromised by a lack of vitamins B2 and B3, copper, iron and coenzyme Q10. These are the ones most immediately involved in its function, although others play a secondary role.

b) Impaired mitochondrial function

The mitochondria need very many different nutrients to function correctly. These include vitamins B1, B2, B3, B5, biotin, manganese, zinc and magnesium. Toxic elements such as mercury, arsenic antimony and fluoride can interfere with mitochondrial functions, as can many other toxins.

3. Toxins and acidic tissues

Almost all books on the CAM approaches to cancer, as well as many of those on other degenerative diseases, will warn of the dangers of toxins. They generally recommend a variety of detox regimes such as improving your diet, drinking vegetable and fruit juices, doing daily enemas and occasional colonic and liver flushes. These and more are described in *Vital Signs for Cancer*.

Other books will tell you that you should be on an alkaline diet and eliminate toxic acid waste material. This is sometimes confusing when you are also told to eat lots of vegetables and fruits that may seem to be acidic, so an explanation is appropriate here. What is meant is a diet that leaves an alkaline residue in the body, not a diet of foods that in themselves are alkaline. This alkaline-residue diet is indeed one that is rich in vegetables and fruits. Even when they are acidic, such as tomatoes or citrus fruits, the residue they leave in the body is largely alkaline, partially due to their high content of essential minerals.

A diet high in proteins (made up of amino *acids*) and fats (made up of fatty *acids*) are not only acidic, but have only trace amounts at best of the alkaline minerals. Even carbohydrates such as sugars and starches generally leave an acidic residue in the body, although the connection with the word 'acid' is less direct. In fact, cancer cells have difficulty using either fats or proteins for energy whereas they thrive on glucose.

Thus, to ensure alkaline rather than acid tissues you should follow a diet in which vegetables and fruits make at least three quarters of the total.

Genetic changes

There are several types of genetic change that follow on from this mitochondrial failure.

Firstly, some existing genes, the proto-oncogenes, that are normally inactive, can be 'turned on'. They can become activated and turned into cancer-promoting oncogenes. Some quiescent oncogenes can also be activated

Secondly, some genes can be altered and can mutate. They then fail to function, or, worse, can block the action they are supposed to support. Thus they can effectively become oncogenes. But remember, these genetic changes are not, as is often claimed, the primary cause of cancer. They are the consequences of the epigenetic changes that damage the electron transport chain and the mitochondria.

These genetic changes can lead to the six features that are the characteristics of cancer, are common to cancer cells, and are an essential part of the development and survival of cancer cells and tumours.

Hanahan and Weinberg have formally proposed the six features that are common to cancer cells and that are an essential part of their development and survival. These are:

- self-sufficiency in growth signals;
- uncontrolled growth;
- the avoidance of growth inhibiting signals;
- avoidance of apoptosis;
- ongoing angiogenesis; and
- metastatic potential.[16, 17]

The first five characteristics are common to benign and to malignant tumours. The characteristic that is unique to malignant cancer cells is the ability to metastasise.

For cancer cells to survive:

1. They must evade differentiation

Differentiation is equivalent to specialisation in which an undifferentiated or non-specialised immature cell develops into a fully differentiated, specialised adult cell, such as a kidney cell, a skin cell or a brain cell. To become cancer cells, undifferentiated, totipotent cells with the potential to divide rapidly into a huge number of daughter cells must avoid specialisation into specific tissue types. Once a cell has started on the process of differentiation and specialisation it is progressively less and less able to divide and multiply, and the ability to divide and multiply is a prime and essential attribute needed by cancer cells. Alternatively, a fully-differentiated cell must dedifferentiate back to a less specialised state, so that it can regain the ability to reproduce daughter cells and can change direction and become a cancer cell.

2. They must evade growth control

All healthy cells obey instructions including the controls that prevent them from multiplying beyond the numbers required by the local tissue for healthy growth, repair and replacement. Potential cancer cells must evade growth inhibiting signals.

3. They must avoid apoptosis

In a healthy nucleus protein53 (p53) monitors each new daughter cell and, if it is found to be faulty, this protein either initiates repair or, if that is unsuccessful, triggers apoptosis. To become a cancer cell each new cell must evade the action of p53. One way in which this occurs is when the p53 gene has become mutated. Cancer cells also rely on there being only limited amounts of BAX (a pro-apoptotic compound) and increased amounts of Bcl-2 (an anti-apoptotic compound). Healthy and normal (non-mutated) p53 stimulates the activity of BAX and hinders the activity of Bcl-2. **All three of these compounds are components of the Second Test Panel and are discussed later.**

4. They must be able to protect themselves from attack by your immune system

Your immune system would normally orchestrate the destruction of foreign or abnormal cells if they did not rapidly die of themselves. A weak immune system is less well able to protect you than is a healthy one. Your immune system depends for its function, on many of the essential nutrients. To protect it you need a nutrient-rich diet. You should also do all you can to avoid other infectious agents and thus overworking this immune system. Many people who develop cancer say, often proudly, that they are never ill and never get a temperature. In fact this is often an indication not of good health but of inadequate immune response.

5. They must develop the capacity to evade attack

Cancer cells are inherently genetically unstable. This gives them great flexibility and they readily adapt to their surroundings and learn to protect themselves. Ironically, one of the disadvantages of chemotherapy is that many of the chemotherapeutic chemicals actually turn cancer cells into cells that become resistant to the drugs. They are then known as Medical Drug Resistant cells (MDR cells).

You may have had chemotherapy, been told that your tumour had reduced in size, even by as much as over 95%, and that you are well on the way to recovery. In all probability you will be thrilled to learn this. However, there are two problems with this. One is that in any tumour only a relatively small percentage of the cells are actually cancer cells, the rest are healthy cells. Many chemotherapy agents can kill off the healthy cells much more rapidly and easily than they can kill the cancer cells. This means that the remainder of the tumour may have a very much higher proportion of cancer cells, cells that are more difficult to destroy by chemotherapy agents or CAM therapeutic agents. Secondly, the use of some chemotherapy agents can actually enable cancer cells to develop *increased* ability to evade attack by this same chemotherapeutic agent.

Survivin is a protein that enables cancer cells to evade attack and to survive. **The survivin gene is one of the genes tested for in the Second Test Panel.**

That is what cancer cells need to survive. Now let's move on to what is required for these cancer cells to develop into a metastatic malignant tumour.

For a cancer cell to develop into a malignant and metastatic tumour and for the tumour to survive it needs:

1. The ability to migrate

For a cancer cell to be able to migrate it has to break out of the original tumour, travel through the extracellular matrix, and then break through the basement layer of the blood vessel wall so that it can then enter and travel through the bloodstream. Many steps are involved in this process. Some of them are aided by enzymes called matrix metalloproteinases (MMPases) which code for proteins with similar names, matrix metalloproteins (MMPs). One of these, **MMP-2, is particularly important, and the gene for this protein is one of the components of the Second Test Panel.**

2. <u>A location to which it can anchor and grow</u>

Anchoring in a new location is a lot more difficult than it may sound. At the new location the cancer cell or cells have to break out of the bloodstream and force their way through the extracellular matrix of the tissue at the destination. This too requires MMPs.

3. <u>A blood supply</u>

Growing tissue needs its own blood supply, one that can reach and nourish each individual cell. To achieve this, new blood vessels need to grow, a process known as angiogenesis. This blood supply is needed to bring nutrients to each cell and disperse waste products. A compound called vascular endothelial growth factor (VEGF) is one of the agents that facilitate this. **The gene that codes for VEGF is a component of the Second Test Panel.**

Genes and Cancer

You may still be wondering if your genes, the components of your genetic inheritance, are not more important than is being indicated here. So we will briefly explore this concept a little further.

In regard to the development of cancer, it is true that your genetic make-up can eventually come into play, or make cancer more likely, but not necessarily inevitable. Cancer will only develop when damage has already been caused within the mitochondria. This damage can come about in many ways.

<u>Genes and enzymes</u>

You now know that genes are the blueprint for the synthesis of proteins and that many of these proteins are enzymes that catalyse most of the thousands of reactions that occur throughout your body. Without these enzymes the reactions that they catalyse would occur so slowly as to inhibit normal healthy function almost entirely.

It is possible that your genetic make-up is such that the production of certain enzymes is below the ideal level and that you do not make them in sufficient quantity or fast enough for optimum function. This may reduce somewhat (but not totally) the efficiency of a certain reaction and so will slow down a specific chemical pathway. This is not ideal, but there are things you can do to improve the situation.

You cannot 'eat' genes, or add them to your diet as supplements. There is a high probability that they would be denatured in your stomach. At best this could mean that they become altered in shape so that they become ineffective and are no longer appropriate blueprints for the synthesis of the desired (protein) enzymes. They could even be broken down within your digestive tract. After all, you probably eat flesh or seeds, with their DNA and genes, every day, but they do not become active in your body.

Even if genes could be absorbed it is unlikely that they would arrive at the specific cells in which they are needed at just the time their actions are needed to facilitate the production of specific protein enzymes. To be fully effective, genes that are active within cells have to be made within the cell where they are required, so that they can stimulate the production of enzymes at precisely the time, often to within fractions of a second, that these enzymes are required. Thus it is generally, though not always, true that you can do little to change your genetic activity in such a way that you change the level of output of these enzymes. However, you can frequently do a lot to improve their efficiency.

Most enzyme catalysts work in conjunction with facilitating partners, known as coenzymes. By definition and common acceptance almost all coenzymes are not made in your body but are, hopefully, delivered as part of a healthy diet.

Many of these coenzymes are either vitamins, usually the water-soluble B group vitamins, plus vitamin C and its cofactors, or the trace elements or minerals such as selenium, magnesium, manganese and zinc. By increasing your intake of these cofactors you can help to improve and optimise the function of the enzymes. By following a diet from which you obtain inadequate amounts of these nutrients, or a lifestyle that interferes with your absorption of these nutrients, you can aggravate the problem. This, in turn, can stress or damage the electron transport chain and the mitochondria.

An enzyme might, for instance, need vitamin B6 as a coenzyme. If you knew this, and knew that your gene that coded for (was the blueprint for) this protein was functioning poorly, you could increase your intake of vitamin B6 and help to compensate for this. Or you may have an increased requirement for chromium, a mineral that is an essential part of the process of normalising the way your body handles glucose. Without chromium, insulin is much less able to transport glucose from your bloodstream into your cells. Had you known this, a diet rich in chromium could have led you to a diabetes-free diet. Your doctor, not trained in nutrition, may not recommend that you take a chromium supplement (along with vanadium and other nutrients in generous amounts), but they should, and a naturopathic or alternative practitioner almost certainly will. When you assist your cells in this way their normal and healthy uptake of glucose will improve and this will help you to maintain normal blood glucose levels and avoid the high blood glucose levels that can increase the risk of cancer.

Countless other similar examples could be given.

Your genes and other proteins

Not all proteins are enzymes. Many of them are structural protein. Examples include those of your muscles, connective tissue and your organs. Others are various types of functional proteins. Some of these are hormones, such as thyroid-stimulating hormone or adrenalin. Others are neurotransmitters. Some play a direct role in the prevention of cancer, such as p53, already mentioned. Again, there are things you can do, with improved diet, nutritional supplements and a variety of nutriceuticals, to compensate for a shortfall in the genes that code for these proteins. This will be discussed in much more detail in the next book in this series, *Targeting Cancer*.

Your genes and freedom

The fact that your genes are not all powerful in predicting your health means you do not need to feel powerless, nor should you. The fundamental cause of the development of the great majority of cancers remains the epigenetic factors that impact on your mitochondria, and you do have control over these epigenetic factors. So keep in mind that in cancer, as in the majority of other degenerative diseases, your genes do come into play, but only as secondary problems caused by harmful epigenetic factors. It is worth repeating: the ultimate cause of cancer is a cellular failure triggered by the epigenetic factors. These cellular changes then act on some of your genes.

There are several outcomes to this and it is now time to explore them.

Not all genes are expressed all the time, nor should they be. It may seem strange that there are genes that code for products that increase the risk of cancer and, once it has started, make it worse. Yet these products do have their purpose, they just have to be kept under control. Some are only active *in utero* and similar times of rapid growth. Some genes are never triggered into action. Some examples will explain this.

You have, for instance, genes that increase the production of a compound called vascular endothelial growth factor or VEGF, one of the components of the Second Test Panel. VEGF encourages increased growth of lots of new blood vessels. This is important, in health, when you have a wound. The new tissues, needed for repair, will need new blood vessels. Thus, when tissue is damaged the gene that codes for VEGF is activated. This is beneficial when new tissue really is needed. In cancer, however, this gene can also be triggered by the cancer cells themselves, and the new blood capillaries are used to supply a blood system that nourishes the growing tumour. The gene does not act of its own volition, but only when triggered by epigenetic factors.

There are other examples. For instance, when the embryo is growing, millions of new cells are needed in a relatively short period of time. It takes only nine months for two minute cells to come together and grow into a seven pound (or more) baby. This is an exceedingly rapid growth rate. It is facilitated by a compound known as carcino embryonic antigen or CEA. **CEA is one of the components of the First Test Panel.** Once the birth weight is reached it is undesirable for this growth rate to continue. CEA production and activity therefore slow down and eventually cease altogether. The gene that codes for it is frequently and inappropriately activated in cancer, stimulating an increased rate of cellular division and reproduction. Arguably this is the result of the carcinogenic epigenetic factors that are part of your lifestyle and diet, and that trigger the initial cellular fault. The growth rate of the tumour is increased by the activity of CEA.

There is one more concept, briefly mentioned earlier, that needs to be brought in here to help to fill out the general picture. You will recall that there are many genes that are known as oncogenes. As their name implies, these are genes that stimulate the various activities that contribute to cancer. It is epigenetic factors that can stimulate these genes into activity. There are also the proto-oncogenes, the genes that can be turned into oncogenes either as a result of mutations (errors of DNA replication) or adverse epigenetic factors. Many epigenetic factors (or carcinogens) can stimulate the conversion of a proto-oncogene into its oncogene form and activity.

So yes, genes do play a role, but not a prime causative role. We will keep coming back to the fact that the prime cause of cancer is the environmentally-triggered cellular faults, at the mitochondrial level, that are triggered by the prime cause, your errors of lifestyle and diet. So you are in control and there is an immense amount of positive input open to you and your prevention and/or recovery. This makes it all the more important that you look after your health, take preventive action and do the various tests, particularly those in the two test panels discussed here, to learn (a) whether or not you are at the earliest stage along the Cancer Process; and (b) what particular approaches you need to take to restore your health.

CHAPTER 6

PRACTICALITIES

Lifestyle and Diet

Remember there is now a large body of research that attributes the cause of cancer to epigenetic factors, and so to your lifestyle, including your diet, and to things over which, to a large extent, you can exert some control. Biava[18] and others[19] put this as high as 93% to 95%. Even conservative UK research has shown that 43% of cancers could be avoided by making just a few sensible decisions around such simple lifestyle factors as those related to smoking, drinking and diet.[20]

These are factors over which you have almost total control. You also have huge control over a wide range of chemicals, now recognised as being potentially harmful, that you personally add to your home and apply to your body. So whatever the figure, there is a huge amount you can do to both prevent cancer and, if you have it, to aid your recovery. As such, it makes sense to get the earliest possible information of any impending problem and make appropriate changes, if that is what is required to prompt you into action. That is at least part of the value of the two test panels proposed here.

If cancer is largely caused by your lifestyle, this also means, if you have cancer, that your own diet and lifestyle choices, in the widest possible sense, have led to you having cancer. So let's get one issue out of the way. This does not mean you are at fault, at least not entirely so, nor does it make you a bad person or mean you are to blame. Many of the features of your lifestyle are dictated by the world in which you live, the regulations laid down by governments and other statutory bodies as to what chemicals are allowed in the marketplace and what industrial practices are permitted. Your choices are probably dictated by the common habits and practices of the community in which you live, the family patterns amongst which you grew up, the pollutants that are allowed to enter the atmosphere and the chemicals that are allowed in the food chain.

You are daily exposed to many chemical and physical toxins, such as atmospheric pollution, chemicals that have been added to and then gradually escaped from materials used in the home and work place, chemicals you are encouraged to use to 'sanitise' your home, and more. Many of these are difficult to avoid. You may have made mistakes, you may have ignored the warnings that are issued daily, about diet, drinking, smoking and chemicals in the workplace, but you have not set out intentionally to harm yourself. You might well argue that you have just done 'what everybody else does'.

Your dietary choices are largely your own, but the various companies and regulatory authorities have decided what is permitted to be included in the food chain. Some ingredients are recognised as carcinogens only after a long period of usage. Farms are allowed to spray toxic chemicals and imbalanced fertilisers, weed killers and pesticides. Other companies are allowed to add countless additives to the foods during processing, such as preservatives, colours, emulsifiers, stabilisers and more. Cosmetic companies are allowed to add a wide range of chemicals to the substances you spread over your skin. Companies are allowed to genetically modify seeds, and we have no idea the extent of the problems that can arise from that practice in the decades ahead. Farmers add antibiotics and hormones to their animals' feeds. All this should stimulate you to consider opting for organically-produced foods and 'natural' cosmetics and household cleaners, made from plant extracts rather than petrochemicals.

Further, emotional issues and stresses play a significant role in developing cancer. Many of the stressors to which you have been subjected may seem to have been outside your control. Others you may knowingly have brought on yourself. The stressors themselves and, even more importantly, the way in which you have reacted to them and dealt with them, can have a major and negative impact on your health.

The list goes on.

All this means that you are 'at cause'. To this extent, you are responsible, but in so far as you did the best you could, you are not to blame. However, once you find out more about the errors of some of these choices, yet do nothing to improve them, then indeed you can truly begin to consider yourself in error for not improving your lifestyle to the extent that you can.

Again, it is worth repeating, exactly because cancer is largely attributable to your total and overall lifestyle, you can, if you wish, make positive changes. There is an immense amount you can do to avoid cancer, if you are willing to minimise your exposure and risk. There is also an immense amount you can do, if you already have cancer, to improve your chances of a recovery. There is much you could have done in the past had you fully understood the risks and the dangers. The past cannot be changed, but it is not too late to start making those changes now. That is why these two test panels are so important. They help to tell you where you are along the Cancer Process, and what corrections you should be making to restore good health.

Other Degenerative Diseases

We can go even further and say that many other serious degenerative diseases also have a large, possibly an overwhelming, diet and lifestyle component as part of their cause. This should come as no surprise. They are, after all, known as degenerative diseases, diseases related to the gradual and progressive degeneration of your body, over time, as a result of the challenges you place on it.

Consider two of the serious diseases that have been hugely on the increase in the last century, heart disease and strokes on the one hand and diabetes on the other. If you suffer from heart problems you may have developed a bad heart, clogged arteries or high blood pressure, but you were not born with a genetically weak cardiovascular system that led inexorably to these problems. After all, heart disease and atheroma-clogged arteries were very rare until as relatively recently as the 1920s. Genetic diseases do not start suddenly and develop this far in less than a century.

You may have developed Type-II diabetes but you were almost certainly not born with a faulty pancreas, or a genetic make-up that decreed that your glucose-handling mechanisms would fail somewhere in mid life. Type-II diabetes was certainly known a century or more ago but it was far less common than it is today.

Again, genetic penetration from a few individuals to such a large proportion of the older members of our population has not proceeded sufficiently rapidly to explain this rise.

Both of these problems have developed largely through lifestyle errors, mainly, but certainly not entirely, those of diet. These two diseases were not nearly so common a century or more ago when we were not exposed to the insults of the toxic chemical world in which we live today and our overly processed and nutrient poor diet.

It is generally recognised, for instance, that eating an excess of overheated and saturated fats, the intake of large amounts of sugars, obesity and lack of exercise can contribute to these problems. Even a nutritionally-reluctant medical profession will generally advocate moderations of diet and lifestyle as part of their treatment plan for both diabetes and cardiovascular problems. This indicates a degree of acceptance of the fact that the correction of causative errors would be helpful in mitigating the problem and restoring homeostasis or general health to the individual.

Cancer and the Medical Approach to Diet – The Anomaly

People with diabetes or heart problems are rarely encouraged to eat fats and sugars, certainly they should not be. It is generally understood, by naturopaths or CAM practitioners, that all types of sugar, in the form of sucrose, glucose, fructose and others, contribute to the risk of the development of diabetes or cardiovascular problems. It is at least recognised by the medical profession that once you have these problems you should reduce your sugar intake and that sugar is a serious risk factor in relation to managing these diseases.

In relation to cancer, the medical profession plays little attention to causes, other than in a very general way. Very few oncologists or medical practitioners consider the causes and how this knowledge could be used in relation to treatment plans. This deserves some comment.

Sugar is, arguably, even more of a risk factor for cancer than it is for heart disease and diabetes. Glucose is the prime fuel that feeds cancer cells. Yet people can have operations to remove malignant tumours, be subjected to radiation or chemotherapy and then be encouraged, by their medical team, the nurses and dieticians, to eat a diet rich in sugar, to 'build themselves up'. This is quite wrong when it is well-researched, demonstrated and proven that glucose is the essential feed for cancer cells. Cancer cells do not thrive on or derive energy from fibre, proteins or fats or a diet rich in vegetables.

It is rare for doctors to advise any dietary improvement in relation to cancer. It is much more common to find that they tell patients not to bother about their diet, that diet has nothing to do with cancer. In fact they generally say that there is nothing whatsoever that you, the individual, can do to help improve your chances of recovering from cancer. This is absolutely wrong. There is an immense amount you can do. You certainly do not need to feel powerless or helpless. Use the results of these tests to help refine your lifestyle and increase your recovery success.

Waiting for Chemo

In case you are tempted to delay making the appropriate positive alterations to your lifestyle, or to delay in doing tests that could give you early warning, or add impetus into your plans to improve your lifestyle, think about the following.

You may be assuming, or have heard via the popular press or from anecdotal stories from people you know, or know of, that chemo, while painful at the time, can offer you a significant chance of recovery if you do get cancer. You may, therefore, be thinking that prevention is not all that vital and that you do not need to do the early warning tests or to make changes to your lifestyle – yet.

A large Australian meta-study into the success of chemotherapy should make you rethink this. A meta-study is one in which the results obtained from a large number of studies are combined so as to rule out misleading results obtained from small sample sizes. They are often used to combine the results obtained from clinical trials of a medical treatment, such as chemo. The Australian study[21] showed that the contribution of chemotherapy to the five-year survival figure of people with cancer was 2.1% in America and 2.3% in Australia. That is very little benefit to very few people at the cost of an immense amount of pain and suffering to almost everyone who received chemotherapy. An Italian study[22] showed a somewhat similar result. In it the use of cisplatin-based therapy, over surgery alone, showed an absolute benefit of only 2.5 to 4.1%.

Do not sit back and think that if you do get cancer you will be able to leave it to the doctors to fix things for you. They won't. It will be up to you.

CHAPTER 7

SUMMARY SO FAR

It is appropriate, at this point, to bring these ideas together. Some of the following may seem repetitive, but it should help to clarify many of the points already made, and possibly add some new ones.

In the conventional medical model it is often stated that cancer results from the action of anything that causes a mutation within the DNA of the nucleus. Such substances are then labelled, by definition, as mutagens. If the mutation does not lead to the destruction of the cell but allows it to evade the normal controls and to reproduce out of control, the cells can grow into a tumour. It is called a benign tumour if it remains localised and does not lead to the creating of metastatic foci elsewhere. Although called benign, it may do significant harm *in situ* simply because of the size to which it can grow and the harmful impact it can have on the local area or the function of the organ or tissue in which it is located. If the mutated gene leads to a cell that not only evades the normal controls and reproduces out of control to grow into a tumour, but leads to the formation of cells that can escape from their starting point and spread to other tissues, the starting insult is recognised and labelled, not only as a mutagen but also as a carcinogen. This is when the tumour becomes truly dangerous.

In the alternative model that we are discussing here the majority of cancers are thought to result from epigenetic factors that lead to damage to, or interference with, the normal function of the energy-producing mitochondria and its electron transport chain, and with the cell's membrane and general cytosol. In other words, if you have cancer, there is thought to have been one or more (almost certainly more) extra-nuclear, external or epigenetic triggers that result from the various Risk Factors, Predisposing Factors and generalised metabolic errors as described in *Vital Signs for Cancer*. These triggers then initiate cellular changes, of undifferentiated stem cells or dedifferentiated mature cells, such that, over time, they become cancer cells.

The importance of this concept is as follows:

If the prime initiating cause of cancer is internal, either inherited genetic aberrations or mutagenic damage to the nuclei of your cells, you have limited therapeutic options. Arguably you are not in control. It is relatively difficult for you to intervene and to alter your genetic make-up or to halt or reverse these genetic changes.

If, on the other hand, it is true that external factors that lead to compromised mitochondrial failure and compromised cell membranes are the fundamental cause of cancer then there is a great deal you can do to help yourself. You can make changes in your lifestyle that help you to both prevent and recover from cancer. You can do this by eliminating any Predisposing Factors and improving the health of these cellular components and the overall chemistry of your cells.

Compromised mitochondria can, in turn, lead to further cellular damage, and this may indeed cause genetic damage. But this latter damage is a secondary cause. This is why a bad diet, for instance, may cause cancer, but reverting to a good or perfect diet may not, on its own, reverse the Cancer Process. For instance, later you will learn that the beneficial p53 protein can prevent cancer by triggering the destruction of faulty cells, as they are produced. But faulty mitochondrial function can lead to the production of mutations of this p53 gene. A test in the Second Test Panel will tell you this. If such a mutation is found you need to do more than improve the factors that led to your cancer. You need to work on correcting your p53. This can be done.

As we go through the following chapters on the suggested test panels you will discover what other tests you can do to learn what your cancer cells are doing most successfully or aggressively and what, as a result, you need to do to block or reverse their progress. How to achieve this outcome, once these test results are available, will form Book IV in this series, *Targeting Cancer*, but in the meantime, and if you have read the first two books in this series, you already know of a great many things you can do, at least to build the foundation of your recovery plan. For the rest, your practitioner should be able to help you.

It is worth repeating: to be able to treat cancer successfully we have to know what it is, what causes it, how it progresses and how it evades all your normal defences. Cancer cells are not all the same. They vary from person to person, even within the same type or location of cancer.

It is important to stress, and keep in mind, the following points:

a) The incidence of cancer has increased dramatically over the last century. For this to be explained by inherited genetic changes alone you have to invoke genetic changes that would have taken millennia to achieve, not simply a few decades.

b) A growing number of researchers consider that, at the most, seven to ten per cent of cancers, possibly even fewer, are the result of inherited genetic errors.[23, 24] It is thought that the remaining 93 or more per cent of cancers are caused by epigenetic factors such as diet, lifestyle and other aspects of the environment. There is nothing else. Toxins, viruses, pathogens, carcinogens, they are all part of lifestyle and environment. They are part of self-selected life situations, selected either proactively or by default. A large number of them are within your control, others you can limit.

c) In *Vital Signs for Cancer* I described cancer as a two phase process. Phase I consists of all the many Predisposing Factors that, in association with Risk Factors (usually things you cannot now change such as a history of cigarette smoking, your sex, age or the number of past pregnancies), are the triggers that constitute the start of the production of active cancer cells. Phase II consists of the developing cancer cells and the eventual growth of a detectable tumour.

d) Since most cancers are caused by outside factors, by substances, activities or changes that occur or are induced in your body by factors that are initially outside your body, you have some, if a varying amount of, control. You have a large measure of control, for instance, over your diet, less over the substances you put on your body or use around your home. You have less control over the pollution to which you are exposed outside your home. This leaves you in a wonderfully powerful position – if you choose to utilise this power. You are in a position of power over what you can do, or avoid, so that you can reduce your risk of developing or worsening cancer. If you already have cancer you can greatly increase your chances of recovery if you choose to make appropriate changes in what you are doing, particularly to those aspects of your lifestyle that you think may have led to you developing cancer in the first place.

e) The epigenetic factors are not only chemical or physical. Stress, plus mental and emotional issues can have identifiable and damaging effects on your body's physiology and chemistry. In the broadest meaning of the word, stress can lead to cancer. Stress or overload may require attention and some rearranging of your life. Resolving mental and emotional issues is within your control. You may not be able to change the outside events that are distressing to you but you can change your emotional response to them. See my book *From Stress to Success* for a full discussion and helpful strategies. This too is a powerful concept in regard to your ability to achieve both prevention and recovery.

You may wonder why a cell's response to adverse external, or exogenous factors, is to turn into a cancer cell. In fact the response is often a successful short-term solution to a problem, even if, in the long term it threatens the survival of the whole organism, the individual, you. If the exogenous trigger is removed soon enough, and corrections applied, arguably the Cancer Process can be halted and even reversed.

This is true, for instance, of the response to stress, as discussed in more detail in *Cancer Concerns* in the chapter on the concepts proposed by Dr Fryda. Dr Fryda states that adrenal exhaustion and the resulting reduction in blood flow to the cells results in reduced cellular oxygen and therefore reduced ability to process cellular glucose. This leads to this glucose being built into large glycogen molecules, made up of thousands of glucose molecules joined together, as a way of 'getting rid of the glucose' that it cannot utilise sufficiently fast, of storing it until such time as it can be processed, as and when the stress is removed and the adrenal function returns to normal. Two things then happen. Firstly the cells turn from healthy aerobic metabolism to unhealthy anaerobic metabolism.[25, 26] In this way they try to compensate for the lack of energy from the compromised mitochondrial citric acid cycle (which needs oxygen) by, at least in the short term, using up some of this glucose more rapidly, but inefficiently and only partially catabolising it. Secondly, this reliance on the cytosol's anaerobic energy production leads to increased cellular reproduction (see the following Chapter Eight, *Your Mitochondria and Cancer*). As a result, when the amount of glycogen becomes too much and the cells are excessively engorged with it, the rate of cellular division enables more new cells to be produced, in which this glycogen can then be stored.

This can be viewed in another way, starting from Warburg's hypothesis as to the ultimate cause of cancer. The original mitochondrial failure and the failure of the respiratory chain backs the system up such that the converting of pyruvic acid to acetyl groups and the processing of these acetyl groups (as mentioned earlier) slows down, there is a build-up of acetyl groups in the cytosol which in turn leads to a build-up of pyruvic acid and then lactic acid, particularly the bad l-lactic acid. This lactic acid in turn also stimulates the rate of mitosis and cellular division. As a result, more cells are available to store more glycogen to continue dealing with the problem of stress-induced adrenal exhaustion and glycogen build up. This is the short-term solution. It will work, and be helpful, as long as the stressors are short lived and the entire situation can be reversed. If the stress is prolonged, or cannot be resolved, the damage will become more difficult to repair.

If the stress is prolonged the adrenal glands become seriously exhausted. This, in combination with any other relevant epigenetic factors, leads to a progressive increase in the number of anaerobic cells that in turn lead to the formation of cancer cells and to one or more tumours, increasing, inexorably, in number and size. The long-term and fundamental solution is to deal with the stress. In addition, Dr Fryda suggests the use of good (d-) lactic acid as is described in *Cancer Concerns*, and restoring normal adrenal function. Cellular oxygen uptake can be increased by the Budwig protocol, also described in *Cancer Concerns*. A decrease in the intake of dietary sugar and refined carbohydrates is of immense value and can further take the pressure off the cells that cannot process this glucose, or only slowly and with difficulty, unless they opt for the escape route of turning into cancer cells. Simply doing these things may not cure cancer but it is certainly an essential part of prevention. Once cancer has started it is also an essential part of reducing the production of new cancer cells and so is a vital component part of any recovery programme.

When these concepts are combined one can see that the fundamental cause of cancer is almost certainly the epigenetic factors that lead to mitochondrial failure, but that the problem is greatly worsened if the individual is under stress.

Several people, including Dr Otto Warburg[27, 28] and Dr Waltraut Fryda[29] have, independently, suggested that cancer is not a disease.[30] By these, and many others, it is claimed that, as in the example above, cancer is an adaptation by the body in its efforts to deal with adverse outside or epigenetic factors. It is caused or aggravated by the efforts made within the cells of your body, as they endeavour to deal with:

a) oxygen deprivation;

b) deficiency of essential nutrients (mostly but not entirely vitamins and minerals) and other substances such as those required by the mitochondria;

c) a lack of protective phytonutrients that would have been part of our inherited diet when it was rich in plant foods;

d) external toxins;

e) pathogenic organisms and viruses;

f) internal toxins;

g) decreased detox ability;

h) poor liver function;

i) excess intake of glucose from starch and sugar, leading to high blood glucose levels;

j) cellular glycogen engorgement;

k) chronic inflammation;

l) radiation, electromagnetic damage and geopathic stress;

m) organ malfunctions, generally due to some or all of the above;

n) stress, in the form of overload, too many demands being made on the body;

o) adrenal exhaustion;

p) emotional stress, particularly of the helpless and hopeless variety where no non-stressful resolution is perceived;

q) mental, emotional and spiritual issues that are not dealt with in harmony.

In this regard, cancer is totally unlike any other health problem. It is in most cases a greater threat to your life. Yet it is also one of the most preventable and, often, provided you are willing to do all that is required, one of the most manageable. Above all, this management is in your hands. Keep in mind that it is not usually the primary tumour that kills you, although a tumour may be so space occupying that it compromises the function of other organs and systems. What usually kills you is the accumulative effects of all the Predisposing Factors that set the full Cancer Process in motion and that continue to fuel it and its metastatic potential.

Finally, it is vital that you keep in mind that once the Cancer Process has started, simply correcting the Predisposing Factors will probably not be sufficient to stop the process. When an object falls off a table and breaks it has to be put back on the table to reverse the situation and recover its position, but additional repair work is also necessary. Simply reversing back out of the Cancer Process via the way you came in, while essential, is generally not enough; you will have additional work to do. For example, considering Dr Fryda's thesis, it is clear that while stress and adrenal exhaustion can cause cancer, simply removing the stress from your life is not sufficient to cure the cancer. The glycogen-engorged cells have been created and they will continue to pump out the harmful l-lactic acid which continues, in its turn, to fuel mitosis and the rapid production of many more cancer cells. You need to take further action to reverse or correct this.

This is why the two test panels, described in the following pages, are so important. They will tell you more precisely what you need to do to aid recovery, over and above removing the causes.

CHAPTER 8

YOUR MITOCHONDRIA AND CANCER

This chapter was originally written as a stand-alone article. As such there is some repetition of preceding chapters, but there is also much that is new; it is written from a slightly different perspective and worth including.

"The cause of cancer is no longer a mystery; we know it occurs whenever any cell is denied 60% of its oxygen requirements."[31]

"Cancer, above all other diseases, has countless secondary causes. But, even for cancer, there is only one prime cause. ...the prime cause of cancer is the replacement of the respiration of oxygen in normal body cells by a fermentation of sugar."[32]

Thus stated Nobel Prize Winner Dr Otto Warburg 90 years ago.

Every time Dr Warburg put healthy cells in a controlled laboratory environment and totally deprived them of oxygen he found that they had turned into cancer cells. They reverted back to being undifferentiated (non-specialised) cells, eminently capable of repeated uncontrolled replications and multiplying to form a tumour. With an adequate supply of oxygen they reverted back to aerobically functioning healthy cells. Modern research continues to prove Warburg's theory.[33]

Warburg postulated that there were several reasons behind these failures:

*   Oxygen deficiency at the cellular level.
*   Deficiency of the nutrients needed for mitochondrial function, what Warburg called the 'essential factors'. Vitamins were only just being discovered in the 1930s and were probably not named in the late 1920s when he was proposing his theory. However, it was obviously known that certain essential factors were needed for correct mitochondrial function. These essential nutrients include at

the most immediate level of involvement: vitamins B1, B2, B3, B5, biotin, CoQ-10, lipoic acid and a number of trace elements. Other nutrient deficiencies can have a more indirect impact on mitochondrial function.

* A wide variety of toxins.
* Emotional issues.

So what are these mitochondria, the failure of or damage to which can lead to cancer?

Your cells consist of a cell wall or membrane, surrounding a fluid but structured cytosol. Within this cytosol, and held in place by a variety of structures, somewhat like scaffolding, are the many different organelles (or organs) of the cell. One type of cell organelle is the mitochondrion.

Mitochondria are unusual organelles, different in several ways from the other organelles within your cells, and it is useful for our purposes, particularly in relation to cancer, but also in relation to other degenerative diseases, to consider them in more detail. To do this we have to go back in time.

There have, over recent decades, been a variety of theories as to how our earliest cells evolved, and there is still discussion and debate on this topic. The following is a current and immensely simplified view, although there are others. Overall, however, it seems clear that mitochondria are 'captured' organisms that 'we', or our earliest single cellular ancestors, engulfed. A much more detailed and very interesting discussion can be found in a book by Lane.[6] However, the following will serve our purpose.

About two billion years ago, long before 'us', there were single-celled organisms, without nuclei, from the archaea group. The archaea were prokaryocytes (cells without nuclei or other organelles) and distinct from the bacteria that existed at the time.

---

[6] Lane, N., *Power, Sex, Suicide*. Oxford University Press, 2005

Living organisms derive energy from the substances they take in, absorb or digest. They use it to convert low energy ADP molecules to higher energy ATP molecules. Think of recharging a battery. ATP is, in effect, the cellular energy currency. This ATP can then be used to drive all the many thousands of reactions that are required to keep the organisms, from bacteria to humans, functioning. Each time ATP supplies its spare energy to a process it falls back to ADP which can then be regenerated to ATP using the energy from the next intake of food or fuel.

All those billions of years ago, when the atmosphere was very different to that of today, archaea derived their energy without the need for oxygen (anaerobically) and produced methane gas as a by-product or waste product.

During the first Ice Age the earth's surface was entirely covered in ice. The level of oxygen in the atmosphere began to rise exponentially and the levels of carbon dioxide and methane decreased significantly. This put the lives of the archaea in jeopardy.

Other single-celled organisms, the proteobacteria, could take advantage of this increase in oxygen and could use it to derive energy from their 'food' and produce energy by oxidative reactions.

In combination, the archaea and proteobacteria could become a significant pair with many survival advantages. It is thought that the archaea absorbed some of these proteobacteria. Within this combination, the archaea component of the cell could thrive and produce ATP when oxygen levels in the atmosphere fell. The proteobacteria component within the cell could thrive and produce ATP when oxygen levels rose. Whether the oxygen level rose or fell, the archaea with its subsumed proteobacteria, now known as a eukaryocyte,[7] could survive. It could produce energy 'whatever the weather'.

These proteobacteria are thought to have evolved into the mitochondria within the cells of all eukaryocytes or, for our purposes, all higher organisms. To this day mitochondria retain many of the

---

[7] Cells with a nucleus.

characteristics of certain types of bacteria, most clearly of the alpha-proteobacteria.[34] They look, in shape and internal structure, for instance, like bacteria. The average human cell now contains around 1,500 mitochondria, whilst neurons, which can be very large cells, are particularly well supplied, often with almost 5,000 mitochondria. The exceptions are your red blood cells. Mature ones have no mitochondria. Their job is to transport oxygen to all your other cells, not use it up themselves.

These mitochondria also retain an element of independence. They have their own genetic material in the form of mtDNA which has some of the characteristics of their ancestral proteobacteria.

This cell combination of archaea and proteobacteria produced ATP in two ways. We will take glucose, the energy fuel derived from virtually all carbohydrates. Within the archaea, now the cytosol of this cell combination, two ATPs can be produced, without oxygen, from every glucose molecule.[8] Within the proteobacteria, now the mitochondria, with the use of oxygen, 36 ATPs can be produced from one molecule of glucose. Clearly the latter is much more efficient. It also propelled us at increased speed, along the evolutionary pathway, since with all that energy the cells could do more and could evolve ever more rapidly.

The ability to produce energy by utilising oxygen[9] was of great benefit, but it also had some disadvantages. During the process of producing energy in this way there is considerable output of super reactive free radicals that can damage the surrounding compounds and tissues. These free radicals could be particularly damaging to the cell's DNA, within the nucleus, so it is fortunate that these reactions now occur within the mitochondria and away from the cell's nucleus. It is one of the reasons why so many 'anti-oxidant' nutrients are need for the maintenance of good health.

A further level of protection for the nuclear DNA was required during mitosis, the process by which two daughter cells (they are never called sons) are being produced. During this time the double stranded

---

[8]   Via the Embden-Meyerhof pathway.

[9]   Via oxidative phosphorylation.

DNA uncoils and 'unzips', thus becoming more vulnerable to free radical damage. It is preferable, during this time of cellular reproduction, to rely on anaerobic energy production.

Thus we have the cytosol producing energy for cell division and for repair and the mitochondria producing energy for cellular function and metabolism. During mitosis and the formation of the new cell, the focus is on the anaerobic form of energy production. After that the focus should move strongly towards full mitochondrial function. In healthy cells the full focus of energy-producing chemistry should be on the mitochondria. If, after mitosis and the formation of the new cell, energy production does not swing back to the mitochondrial method, cellular integrity can be compromised and the cell can become damaged. Healthy, oxygen-rich, mitochondria, as Dr Otto Warburg hypothesised, are required for good health. If these mitochondria are damaged in any way, poor health, at both the cellular level and the level of the total organism, will result.

Modern research, supporting the near century old hypothesis of Warburg, demonstrates that a lack of the essential nutrients and anti-oxidants, needed for mitochondrial function can damage the mitochondria.

There are two aspects of energy release (from food components) within the mitochondria. These are first the citric acid cycle. During this, energy is released from the starting material in the form of very high energy molecules. These have too much energy for normal cellular reactions. It would be a bit like using the full force of a blast furnace to warm a small sitting room. The second phase within the mitochondria is known as the respiratory chain or the electron transport chain. During this chain of reactions the energy is released from the very high energy compounds and used to convert several molecules of ADP into several of slightly higher ATP.

Several essential nutrients are needed by the electron transport chain, and without them the membranes of the mitochondria can become blocked. As a result, the entry and exit channels within the mitochondrial membrane cannot function; the mitochondria neither take in oxygen or essential nutrients nor export ATP, other compounds or waste products.[35] If this leads to a build-up of those dangerous free radicals, significant destructive damage can also be caused.

The cellular self-protecting response to this is to reduce mitochondrial energy-generating activity, and lead to greater cellular reliance on the cytosol's anaerobic energy-producing pathway. However, this should only be the major source of energy during tissue repair and cellular reproduction. Not only is this strategy inefficient as a source of energy, it also encourages cellular reproduction.

Thus, mitochondrial failure or damage can lead to chronic exhaustion. It can also lead to a variety of other and more serous degenerative diseases. Worse, this focus on increased and excessive cellular reproduction is an obvious characteristic of cancer cells. Otto Warburg, with little knowledge of what we now know about mitochondrial function, seems to have been amazingly perceptive and ahead of his time.

A lack of oxygen can block mitochondrial function and move the energy focus to the anaerobic cytosol with its greater stimulus for increased cellular production. This happens in a variety of ways, not only due to damaged DNA but to increased output of lactic acid which is one of the consequences of this reaction sequence. A lack of his 'essential factors' or as we now know them, essential vitamins and trace elements, can cause failure at the level of the electron transport chain. There are many toxins that can cause similar problems, as can the consequences of stress, particularly prolonged and unresolved stress. But that is a further story.

It also seems that not all ATP is created equal. Cytosol ATP is a much simpler molecule, at the atomic level, than mitochondrial ATP, for reasons we won't go into here. Mitochondrial ATP is, for instance, an important signalling molecule. A reduction in the amount of this ATP is damaging to the cell in many ways. For instance it has an important relationship to inflammatory reactions and inflammation is a contributing factor to cancer.

So, the prime cause of cancer is mitochondrial damage, triggered by many *outside* or epigenetic factors, such as poor diet, nutrient deficiencies and the presence of toxins. This damage can lead to many problems, including fatigue and failures at all levels of your body. It can trigger damage to the cell's DNA, to genetic mutations, some of which can trigger cancer. Genes may *seem* to be causing cancer, but except in rare cases, they are *not* the primary cause.

Since the primary cause is external to you, part of your lifestyle and diet, you have an enormous weapon you can use in your attempts to either prevent or recover from cancer. Change and improve your lifestyle and diet.

You are not your genes. You are the result of the lifestyle you choose and the effects this has on you mitochondria and hence on your genes. Good genes can be activated by a healthy lifestyle. Genes that should only be active, during the very active growth period *in utero*, and genes that are inherently oncogenes[10] can lie quiet, all your life from birth onwards. Or they can be triggered by toxins, nutrient deficiencies, lack of cellular oxygen and mitochondrial damage.

The millions of dollars or pounds, raised by well-meaning individuals, charities and related organisations, and used for research into the genetic causes of cancer, may provide useful funds for genetic research. It may provide income for the various drug companies that focus on developing products to impact on genetic changes or tumour destruction. But it does little to help people with cancer.

It would be of enormously much greater benefit, to people suffering from cancer, if these funds were put to use improving our environment, removing or reducing the enormous load of toxins to which people are daily exposed, and encouraging people to adopt a better lifestyle and improve their diet. This may not sound as exciting as new high-tech equipment methods of destroying tumours, or exciting new drugs with their toxic consequences, but it would be a lot more effective. Putting more research money into furthering our understanding of mitochondrial function, and the failure of this function, in relation to cancer, and ways to prevent or remedy this failure, would almost certainly be a more helpful path to follow.

---

[10] Genes whose activity leads to cancer.

CHAPTER 9

THE TESTS

Now that you understand the nature of your cells, the Cancer Process, and the changes that occur as they change from healthy cells to cancer cells, and the effect of epigenetic factors, it is time to talk about how you can use this information.

Early Detection

For a large proportion of the time, during which the Cancer Process is developing, the process goes undetected. It is probable that the first outward and obvious symptom you get will be a lump, a bleed or a cough. By the time this symptom develops the process will have been active for a long time, possibly months but more probably years. During those years, had you known about it, you could have become actively involved in stopping its progression and reversing back to good health. The longer you delay the more difficult this becomes.

What are required are one or more tests that can give you this very early warning. Ideally, these tests should be non-invasive, non-harmful and include your whole body. They should also be reasonably inexpensive and not time-consuming.

Cancer is a systemic problem, not a local one. Phase One can start in cells anywhere in your body, possibly in a wide range of cell types. Phase Two, that of fully-developed cancer cells, is usually more localised but can start almost anywhere. Thus, an overall and systemic chemical test is required if you want to detect cancer early.

There are three aspects of early detection. The first is to detect the problems of Phase One and the presence of, and damage being done by, the various Predisposing Factors. This is discussed below under Preliminary Tests. The second is to detect the start of Phase Two and this is covered by the First Test Panel. The third is to discover the aspects of your particular cancer cells that will enable you to design your recovery programme, and to do so, possibly, long before a detectable tumour has formed. This is covered by the Second Test Panel.

Before we discuss the three groups of tests, there are some other topics to be considered.

Tumour Markers

You may be thinking that the medical approach offers cancer markers, or tumour markers, for early detection and you may be wondering what the difference is between them and the tests described here. There are several very significant differences.

The medical tests for tumour markers do not constitute very early warning tests. They give you too little information too late. They do not, in any way, substitute for the Preliminary Tests. They cannot. By definition they are detecting tumours, not the start of the Cancer Process. By the time you have a tumour you are well into Phase Two of the Cancer Process. The results of the Preliminary Tests described below can warn you that you could be at increased risk of developing fully cancerous cells, Phase One of the Cancer Process. If you take remedial action at this stage you could avoid cancer altogether. Tumour markers cannot help you to do this.

The medical tumour markers are proteins shed from a developed tumour. Thus the tumour *has* to be there *before* the markers are detected. They are useful for testing for the presence of an established tumour, but the detection occurs too late if you want to recover your health and to do so relatively easily. By the time a tumour has formed and is shedding its markers, cancer is already well developed and recovery is more difficult.

Different proteins are produced by different types or locations of tumours. The tumour markers shed by tumours in the breast, ovaries or colon, for instance, are different from each other. So to cover all the possibilities, a blood sample would have to be analysed for many different markers, possibly for markers from every type of tissue throughout your body, if they existed, certainly from as many different tissues as possible.

It is even worse, however. Not all tumours shed readily identified cancer markers. For this reason many tumours cannot be detected in this way.

The First Test Panel deals with these problems. As you will discover, the results of this panel can enable you to detect cancer, systemically, and, arguably, anywhere in the body, within weeks of the formation of the first cancer cells and often months or even years before a tumour develops. Thus, in no way do tumour markers substitute for the First Test Panel.

Another benefit of the First Test Panel is that the results will indicate the extent to which anaerobic metabolism in the cytosol has increased at the expense of healthy aerobic metabolism in the mitochondria. Thus, the results can indicate directions to be taken by the recovery plan. Tumour markers do not do this.

A criticism of this First Test Panel, if the results are positive for cancer, might be that it does not identify the location of the cancer cells. However, this is not necessarily a problem if you are not focused on tumour destruction, as is the medical approach. Once you recognise that cancer is a systemic disease and that recovery will depend on restoring the whole system to normal health, you recognise that the recovery plan will be relatively independent of the location of the tumour.

A claim made for the medical tumour markers is that they do help to indicate the location of the tumour(s). These tumour marker tests tend to be somewhat organ or tissue specific. However, the correlations are neither consistent nor absolute. For instance, CA19-9 is suggestive of cancer of the pancreas, but it could also indicate colo-rectal cancer; CA-125 is suggestive of ovarian cancer but it could also be due to cancer of the lungs or breast.

Finally, tumour markers do little to help you establish the best recovery plan. The Second Test Panel, on the other hand, does just that. By determining the levels of activity of a variety of genes and proteins you gain the information that can help to establish just what is needed to correctly target the characteristics of the cancer. These results will indicate the course a recovery plan should take.

Tumour markers can be used to help monitor treatment after you have developed cancer and have one or more tumours. However, even here, the test panels fare better. If they are repeated, over time, the results you obtain can tell you not only whether or not your recovery is proceeding correctly, but also in what ways you should adjust your actions and modify what you are doing, to obtain the best possible results.

Research Funds and Current UK Legislation

You may wonder why, if the tests suggested here and the CAM protocols suggested for recovery are so effective, your doctor is not using them and why there are only limited trials as to the results they achieve.

A partial answer is that there is little or no money to be made from helping people to improve their diet and lifestyle (see the discussion of Béchamp's view, in the thesis below). It is not possible to patent, and so make money from, specific foods or nutrients. There is, on the other hand, an immense amount of money to be made from patented drug medicine (see Pasteur's view, in the thesis below). Financially, there is a huge vested interest in maintaining the current medical, tumour-focused, approaches to cancer.

It is also possible, via the well-meaning efforts of the many charities involved, to raise large amounts of money for research into all sorts of studies into the activity of specific enzymes or genes that might have a role to play in cancer. This may be wonderful for the research scientists and help to fund university research. It may line the profits of the big drug companies, and the suppliers of the technology of the equipment used in oncology units. It is of doubtful benefit to the people suffering from cancer. This is evidenced by the vast amount of money and research that has gone into the drug approach to cancer over the last several decades with very little increase in survival time (noted above), possibly a worsening rather than an improvement in the quality of life, and little reduction in the incidence of cancer.

This is not a book about the politics of cancer; there are many of those around, most of them very well researched. But it should be obvious, from the increased rate of the disease, that the present medical approach to cancer is not working. The current American statistic, depending on which source you read, is that an individual has a fifty per cent chance of developing cancer at some time in their life. In the UK the figure is put nearer to forty per cent, but in both countries the percentages are rising. If the incidence is increasing, the focus on prevention and very early detection becomes all the more important.

The alternative approach, discussed here, into the nature of the development of the disease, its early detection and its possible reversal, offers many benefits. At the very least it is non-toxic and non-harmful, but it offers a great deal more. It offers the individual a measure of control over their own destiny. It leads, especially via the appropriate use of the test results, to the planning of a rational recovery protocol. It also leads to improved overall general health, individual wellbeing and energy.

Secondly, there is an irony in the current legislation. Currently UK law decrees that no one should claim or imply that they can treat cancer, although this is of course ignored by medical doctors and oncologists. This law can, however, be used against medical doctors who do prescribe complementary or alternative methods for their patients. It can also be used against alternative or CAM practitioners if they make such a claim or advertise that they can treat cancer.

Why is this? Is it because the alternative CAM approach offers significant competition to the drug medicine? If modern medicine was so sure that it had all the answers it would surely show this with improved results. Nor would there be such a groundswell of people choosing to adopt complementary or even alternative options, options that they have seen offer benefits to other sufferers.

This whole topic highlights a difference between the medical and the CAM approach. In the medical approach it is cancer that is the focus and that is treated, specifically it is the tumour on which the focus is placed. In the CAM approach it is the whole person that is treated. Normal homeostasis is the goal. If this is achieved, cancer cannot exist in the body. So in fact CAM therapists do *not* treat cancer, they treat people.

However, this UK law does put people suffering from cancer, or keen to prevent cancer, at a significant disadvantage. It reduces their individual freedom, their ability to find a practitioner of choice that can focus on the problem that concerns them, cancer. It could be argued that this is discriminatory.

At the time of writing there are proposals being put before the UK parliament to 'allow' doctors to offer some complementary or alternative treatments in certain situations. The details have yet to be debated. However, this may mean that doctors are only 'allowed' to recommend CAM protocols, which can readily run alongside medical treatments if the individual so chooses, when conventional medical methods have failed, and if a panel of medical doctors agree that this should be done. It could be seen as a hopeful step forward, but only a very small one. Currently there are many doctors who would like to offer such alternative treatments, either alone or in conjunction with the medical options, but who know they risk censure from their medical colleagues and possible loss of their licence if they do so.

Tests, Their Value and Reliability

It is time to move forward and consider the various tests you can do to help you prevent, detect and monitor the possible start of both Phase One and Phase Two of the Cancer Process.

An immediate question could be: are these laboratory tests absolutely necessary? No, if funds are short you can do without the very early warning tests, as long as you focus on including all the lifestyle changes and dietary improvements that are required for optimum health. However, few people are willing to do this, preferring instead to ignore the warnings and types of advice that are available. It is too easy to assume that it 'won't happen to me'. Given the odds, this is false optimism. Most people are only willing to make significant changes in their life when they have been triggered (frightened?) into this by some early warning test results.

What about when cancer has already been confirmed? You could choose not to do the Second Test Panel. You might choose instead to include in your recovery plan, in addition to improving your lifestyle and diet and detoxing, all the remedies that have been suggested for helping to restore your health when you have cancer. However, this is something of a shotgun approach. If you can target your actions, based on the results of the tests discussed here, not only can it lead to a more successful outcome, it could also save you money, in the long run, on the remedies that you may not need.

If funds are really short you can focus on dietary improvements such as determining your Metabolic Type and following the diet as indicated by the results of this test, and including the suggestions of Dr Kelley and Dr Budwig. All of these were discussed in *Cancer Concerns*. However, if you follow that route and then later do the tests discussed below you may find you are, or have been, eating some unhelpful foods and failing to include in your diet some foods that would have been highly beneficial. You may also find you are, or have been, taking some supplements you do or did not need and omitting others that could have made a significant difference. In the long run, doing these tests can help to focus your efforts and make them more successful.

False negative and false positives

Few medical or physiological tests are perfect. The functioning of the human body is too complex for that. There are almost always some false negative results, where detection is missed, or false positive results where a problem is thought to exist when in fact it does not. Before planning a testing protocol, it is important to understand these facts in relation to the tests being performed, the use that will be made of the results, and the possible consequences of any such errors.

Where do you want to draw the line? Do you want to minimise the risk of missing a diagnosis, even if that means increasing the risk of a false positive diagnosis? Or do you want to be sure that all the positives really are positive (in this case bad) signs, even if that means getting a false negative result and missing a diagnosis?

In this regard it is important to keep in mind that the dominant component cause of cancer is made up of your lifestyle errors. The extent to which this applies ranges from ultra-conservative estimated figures of around 60 per cent to some well-researched figures that places it as high as 95 per cent.[36, 37] This being the case, correction of lifestyle, including diet, should be the dominant focus of any recovery or correction plan. Such changes are most certainly not harmful, and so instigating them does not expose you to the risk of toxic and harmful side effects. In fact, any side effects will be beneficial as you work towards achieving homeostasis and optimum health.

In a healthcare system that aims at restoring normal function by methods that are beneficial to the body and in harmony with its normal and healthy function, not only are toxic effects avoided, but a false positive result is less of a problem than a false negative result. At worst a false positive result can trigger some anxiety, but equally it can be a trigger for you to improve your diet and lifestyle, and could almost certainly improve your general health, even if you do not have cancer. This point is so important that it warrants repetition here. In this situation, it is more important to focus on the avoidance of false negative results and the failure to detect early signs of the problem and so to fail to take preventive measures, than to be too concerned about aiming to avoid a false positive diagnosis.

In a medical system that applies treatments such as surgery, chemotherapy and radiation, all of which have high levels of risk and adverse and toxic effects, up to and including the triggering of cancer itself, it is important to avoid tests that can give false positive results, such as mammograms. It is absolutely suggested, here, that you do NOT instigate any of these potentially toxic medical treatments based solely on the results of the test panels described here. You absolutely can, and should, however instigate alternative, non-toxic and health-inducing protocols and lifestyle changes.

It is for this reason that a panel of tests is suggested, rather than the use of a single test. By using the several tests indicated in the First Test Panel it can be argued that you increase the risk of getting a false positive result, but you also reduce the risk of a false negative, and of missing the earliest possible warning sign.

Bearing in mind that the results of such tests may well be the earliest sign of cancer, a seemingly false positive result, suggestive of cancer, but unconfirmed by other tests, could merely be due to the fact that the indicated test result is indeed the first sign of possible cancerous changes, not yet detectable by less sensitive tests, and not at all 'false'.

It is also pertinent to point out that doing these tests only involves the prick of taking a blood sample and the collection of early morning urine. There are no adverse side effects to these processes. This is in contradistinction to many medical tests such as mammograms and biopsies, which can themselves cause further problems and even cancer itself.

The following tests are divided into three groups. There are those of the Preliminary Tests, the First Test Panel and the Second Test Panel.

CHAPTER 10

PRELIMINARY TESTS

Preliminary tests for detecting Phase One of the Cancer Process should include tests for the many Predisposing Factors. This means tests for:

* the appropriate diet for each individual, according to their metabolic type;
* nutrient deficiencies;
* digestive and liver problems;
* the presence of toxins;
* adrenal exhaustion and states of stress;
* immune dysfunction;
* functional imbalances of blood glucose levels;
* hypothyroidism;
* oestrogen levels;
* other glandular or hormonal failures;
* neurotransmitter imbalances.

These preliminary tests should cover different aspects of diet, nutrition, toxins and individual organ problems. These tests will not tell you whether or not you have cancer. They will tell you whether or not your health is sub-optimal and could be leaving you increasingly vulnerable to the development both of cancer and of other degenerative diseases. A number of laboratories offer a variety of tests within this spectrum and your practitioner should be able to help you with this. These preliminary tests are valuable and important for several reasons.

Firstly, the initial development of cancer occurs at the sub-microscopic level and so is difficult to detect except by blood or urine tests. It is rarely detected by a physical examination at this stage. Thus, early chemical tests for minor but significant physiological and chemical changes are of immense value.

Secondly, you cannot predict where cancer will start so you do not know where to look for early signs when doing a physical search. Chemical tests that relate to fundamental changes in cellular function, on the other hand, can cover your entire body. They can tell you it is somewhere in your body, though not where.

Thirdly, since the changes that lead to cancer are systemic, you can get very useful information from testing at the cellular level. It is a bit like testing the integrity of a building by testing the fundamental state of the building components, the bricks. You don't have to test each wall or room.

Doctors, who focus their treatments almost entirely on the tumour and its eradication, need to wait until there is a tumour large enough to be detected and its location pinpointed. CAM practitioners who take a systemic and holistic approach to the whole body do not need to focus on tumour location. They are not tumour-focused. They can work immediately the earliest possible warning sign is detected to improve your overall body chemistry, metabolism and function, and restore normal homeostasis.

Predisposing Factors are not really a part of this book. They were discussed in detail in *Vital Signs for Cancer*. Nonetheless, the first thing for you to do if cancer is suspected, or if you have been diagnosed with cancer, is to check for any of these factors. Any of them could have triggered the cellular changes and contributed to the epigenetic challenges. Removing these Predisposing Factors from your life and correcting the various errors that are indicated has to be a part of the foundation of your recovery protocol as well. Then, once this is in place and you are no longer encouraging the formation of new cancer cells, it is time to move on. This is the first layer of your recovery programme. It is essential that these Predisposing Factors be corrected.

There is a useful overarching urine test, described below, that can give you a generalised view of your cellular function, even before there are significant changes from healthy cells to cancer cells: The Optimum Nutritional Evaluation or ONE test.

It is important to remember that cancer starts with changes at the cellular level and particularly with changes in mitochondrial function. For this reason it is important to establish the state of the reactions that relate to both overall cellular function and, more specifically, to mitochondrial function. Thus, an important early test should focus on the state of cellular and mitochondrial function. This is the focus of the ONE test offered by Genova Diagnostics. Similar tests may well be offered by other companies and such availability can vary over time, so search around for what is available.

The results of this test can tell you about the level of anaerobic chemistry going on in your cells, whether or not that is raised above normal, and something about the possible causes. Excessive anaerobic cellular function can increase the likelihood of cancer.

In this test the levels of the major components of the citric acid cycle are measured. Remember, this is the cycle of reactions that takes place in the mitochondria and is fundamental to its functioning. Errors in this cycle can suggest that you are at least in Phase One of the Cancer Process, the phase that leads up to the formation of cancer cells. You may also be in Phase Two when cancer cells have formed and reproduced themselves.

The results obtained can lead to a planned nutritional supplement programme. This is because the majority of the reactions within this cycle are facilitated by enzyme catalysts, most of which require several coenzymes. Remember, enzymes are produced according to the instructions that come, eventually from your genes. Coenzymes are the substances that you obtain from your diet, and so over which you do have control. The better your diet and, if you have one, your supplement programme, the better will be the availability of these coenzymes and therefore the functioning of your citric acid cycle. If certain steps of the citric acid cycle are not functioning efficiently you could be deficient in the related cofactors or coenzymes. The test results will tell you this and you can then change or supplement your diet accordingly.

Because so many of the vitamins and minerals required by the body are required by all the various aspects of this nutritional evaluation, including but not limited to, the citric acid cycle, the results can provide useful overall information as to the many of the vitamins and minerals in which you may be deficient.

It is important to emphasise that this nutritional evaluation is not a test for cancer. However, it is an immensely useful foundation or preliminary test if you are interested in determining how your cells are functioning in regard to their basic cellular tasks.

The information gleaned from this test is distinct from tests that provide information as to the cells' specialised activities. The test does not, for instance, measure the effectiveness of your muscle cells at producing muscle contractions and relaxations, the efficiency of lung cells in taking up oxygen, of glandular cells at producing their hormones, or the effectiveness of your liver cells at producing the various compounds that are specific to the unique and complex activities of your liver. What the test does measure, monitor and indicate is valuable information about fundamental cellular activity throughout almost all the cells of your body.

The results will tell you:

a) how effectively you are absorbing the foods that you eat;
b) the possible presence of pathogenic organisms such as clostridia, pseudomonas, *Candida albicans*, or general yeasts;
c) the level of lactic acid and the ratio of it to pyruvic acid and hence the possibility of an increase in adverse anaerobic metabolism;
d) about possible blocks to the Pivotal Point (discussed in *Cancer Concerns*) between pyruvic acid in your cells' cytoplasm and the acetyl groups that enter the citric acid cycle;
e) the levels of the various compounds in the aerobic citric acid cycle within your mitochondria;
f) if there are faults or blockages within your citric acid cycle;
g) how efficient is your fatty acid metabolism, as indicated by a number of ketones;
h) about a range of organic acids, the presence of which can indicate a variety of nutrient deficiencies;
i) about possible metabolic acidosis;

j) about possible protein deficiencies;

k) about possible vitamin deficiencies;

l) about possible mineral deficiencies;

m) about a possible biotin deficiency – common in candidiasis and dependent on a healthy intestine;

n) about the presence of possible carcinoid tumours in the intestinal tract;

o) the level of activity of certain neurotransmitters;

p) about the possible presence of certain neurotransmitter metabolites, which reflect on overall function;

q) the possible presence of certain heavy metal toxins (such as antimony, arsenic, lead, mercury);

r) about xenobiotic toxicity in general;

s) if there is a possible pancreatic deficiency – especially when assessed in conjunction with other tests;

t) about the possibility of kidney stones;

u) about the possibility of hypothyroidism;

v) about possible oxidative stress;

w) warnings in relation to cardiovascular disease.

The report you receive, after doing this test, will normally provide you with the results themselves plus a discussion as to their meaning and indications. In addition you will normally receive suggestions as to possible supplements and remedies that may help you to correct each of the abnormal results that are found, along with suggestions as to confirmatory tests that could add to the clarity of the overall picture.

This is clearly a test that can pick up a lot of the Predisposing Factors and early warning signs. As such, it can help you to tell whether or not you are in Phase One. I have never known anyone to have no errors in the components measured by this test. Correcting any of the errors found will help you to maintain good health and prevent the development of cancer.

This test is also of value if in other tests you have been diagnosed with cancer and are in Phase Two of the Cancer Process. Correcting the errors found by such an extensive test as this will improve your basic cellular function and will constitute a foundation for the rest of your recovery protocol. In other words, everything else you do will work very much better if you correct the foundations of your cellular function, and this test will give you a large measure of the information you need to enable you to do this.

This test is done on a urine sample and so can be sent to the laboratory by post.

CHAPTER 11

THE FIRST TEST PANEL

The First Test Panel aims to help you detect the very earliest possible sign of the start of Phase Two of the Cancer Process. This is the phase where fully cancerous cells have formed and persisted. There may not yet be a detectable tumour, but there is cancer activity at the cellular level. According to the laboratory that does the majority of the tests that make up this panel, these tests are capable of detecting this activity as early as six weeks after the first cancer cells are formed and long before there is a tumour to shed markers. The compounds tested for apply to all the cells throughout the body so it is a comprehensive systemic test.

Keep in mind that a tumour doesn't suddenly occur overnight. There is a long process of reactions and cellular changes that have probably been on-going for several years before the tumour is finally of a sufficient size that it can be discovered. This being so, tests that can detect this process at such an early stage will enable actions to be taken that provide the greatest possibility of recovery. The medical profession looks for ways of finding the tumour as early as possible, so that it can proceed with its damaging, destructive and toxic procedures of surgery, chemotherapy and radiation. The aim here is to look for the start of the preceding process with the aim of gently restoring homeostasis.

One of the boasts of the medical profession is that early detection of a tumour leads to longer survival. But even working to find the tumour earlier is still too late and this is rarely helpful in the long term. The tests that help to find the tumour somewhat earlier may lead to a situation where the individual starts chemotherapy or radiation earlier, and survives for longer from detection to death. However, a number of studies have suggested that this may only be by an increase of time equivalent to the extra length of time covered by the earlier detection. In other words, if you discover a tumour one year sooner than you might have done you might only have an increase in survival time from diagnosis of one year. You have lived for the same length of time but have known about it for longer. If the adverse effects of chemotherapy or radiation are taken into account, these may even shorten your lifespan.

However, and this is a hugely significant point, the story is very different if you are following naturopathic or alternative options. CAM options do not have harmful or carcinogenic toxic or side effects; they are all aimed at restoring homeostasis. Keep in mind that CAM interventions are aimed at restoring normal, healthy cellular function, at removing the carcinogenetic epigenetic factors, at detoxing the body and supplying it with all the nutrients it needs to optimise healthy genetic function, and more.

Because cancer is a process it can be detected by the presence of factors that encourage this harmful process, produced and secreted by the various cells, and found in blood or urine. These factors, the components of the two panels of tests described below, can be analysed for and their correction monitored. Further, this can be done by safe means and positive outcomes achieved even before a tumour is detectable. If you already have cancer these same tests can be used to monitor any recovery protocol you put into place, a protocol that restores normal health, not one that aims to blitz the tumour(s) with little or no regard for collateral damage.

The proposed First Test Panel consists of:

lactic acid
PHI
HCG
TK1
telomerase
CEA

In practice these tests are done by different laboratories (see Appendix for laboratory details). PHI, HCG (3 forms), TK1 and CEA are offered by American Metabolic Laboratories as part of their CA profile. Telomerase is offered by the Galkina Laboratory in the UK. Lactic acid is a component of the Optimum Nutrition Evaluation (ONE) test done by Genova Diagnostics.

Lactic Acid

All the starches and sugars you eat as part of a normal diet are eventually broken down, absorbed and travel through your bloodstream as glucose. This glucose is converted to pyruvic acid in the anaerobic cytosol of your cells. If your mitochondria become compromised the pyruvic acid can no longer enter them, and so it has nowhere to go. As a result it is converted, in a sideways shunt, into lactic acid. This lactic acid cannot be processed within the cells, whether they are cancer cells or healthy cells. Instead it has to travel through your bloodstream and go to your liver, where it is converted back into glucose.

The relatively small amount of lactic acid produced when you exercise or use muscles faster than they can get sufficient oxygen to supply the increased demand on mitochondrial function is not a long-term problem. The on-going and significant production of lactic acid produced by cancer cells is a significant problem.

Measuring your blood level of lactic acid is one part of the First Test Panel.

Not only does a chronic, or long term, increase in your blood lactate level suggest the possibility of cancer, it also encourages it. Lactic acid increases mitosis or cellular reproduction, it increases angiogenesis or the production of the new blood vessels needed for a growing tumour, it helps the cancer cells to avoid immune reactions that could destroy them, and it facilitates metastasis.

Thus, a chronic or persistent increased level of lactic acid increases the aggressiveness of the cancer and indicates a poor prognosis. It also makes the cancer more resistant to any radiation treatment that you may choose.

PHI

Cancer cells need energy, and this is normally provided by the breakdown of carbohydrates, fats and amino acids largely in the mitochondria. If Phase Two of the Cancer Process is active the associated mitochondrial failure will significantly reduce this energy production in the affected cells. They normally obtain less than ten per cent of their energy from reactions within the cytosol. However, to compensate for their energy loss from the mitochondria they increase the first part of glucose breakdown, the Embden-Meyerhof pathway in the cytosol, converting increased amounts of glucose to pyruvate and then lactic acid. To achieve this they increase the production of the enzymes that are required to catalyse the reactions in this sequence. One of these enzymes is phosphohexose isomerase or PHI.

Measuring your blood level of PHI is another part of the First Test Panel.

A chronic increased level of PHI in a serum sample suggests that there is increased activity of the Embden-Meyerhof pathway and so increased anaerobic metabolism with its associated potential for increased production of lactic acid, for mitosis or cell replication, and thus an increased likelihood that cancer is operative.

Not only is PHI indicative of an increased likelihood of cancer, like lactic acid, it also encourages cancer. The alternative name for PHI is AMF or autocrine motility factor, which is discussed further in Section II of this book. The name AMF was given initially as it is produced within the cells (autocrine) and stimulates the motility or movement of the host cells. A raised level of PHI does several things that encourage cancer. It:

- increases the ability of the cells to migrate;
- increases the ability of cells to proliferate;
- inhibits apoptosis;
- stimulates angiogenesis;
- stimulates metastasis.

Thus it increases the ability of cancer cells to survive, to invade and to ensure their own blood supply. Keep in mind that it is the ability of the cells of an otherwise benign tumour to metastasise that converts the benign tumour into a malignant tumour and so suggests a poor prognosis for the individual.

From One Cell to Many

The next component of the First Test Panel is a hormone called human chorionic gonadotropin (HCG), which we will cover next. To understand its role, and the reasons why it is an important component of this test panel some further background information is pertinent.

This next stage was described in some detail in *Cancer Concerns*. It relates to the similarities between the early development of the growing embryo in pregnancy and the development of cancer cells and their growth into a tumour.

Dr John Beard, in around 1905, showed that placental tissue and cancerous tissue were the same. That's right, the same, not similar but identical. In fact, the chemical changes that occur in the embryo in the uterus in the first 55 days of pregnancy are similar to those that occur in the development of cancer.

Very soon after conception the two uniting cells, ovum and sperm cell, grow into a small cluster of about sixteen cells, called the morula. This constitutes the growing embryo. To survive and be successful these cells have to latch onto the uterine wall and avoid being swept away, to penetrate and become embedded in the uterine wall, to avoid attack from the mother's immune system, to multiply rapidly to achieve a secure start in life and to develop access to the mother's blood supply. These processes are essential for its survival. They are difficult, and they require a number of vital chemical and physiological steps if the embryo is to survive. They are also essentially the same as the processes that are required by cancer cells if they are to survive, reproduce and grow rapidly, metastasise to a new location, become established there and continue to grow.

If the uterine process continued without being stopped the embryo would become so large and so dangerous for the mother that she would develop choriocarcinoma or the cancer of pregnancy and both she and the embryo could die. What stops the process is the start of the activity of the embryo's pancreas. At less than two months into the pregnancy the embryo does not need a pancreas to either help in digestion or manage blood glucose level, the two major pancreatic functions. However, it does need the pancreas to produce the pancreatic enzymes that can stop these initial cancer-like functions of the placental cells (or trophoblastic cells).

HCG

One hormone is vital for the processes that facilitate the embryo's ability to attach to the uterine wall, invade it and acquire what it needs from this new location. It is called human chorionic gonadotropin or HCG. It is an essential part of pregnancy. It is also common in many cases of cancer. It is almost never produced by any other cells and so is not detected in the blood of people who are neither pregnant nor have cancer.

HCG is a component of the First Test Panel.

HCG is a complex molecule. As discussed in Section II of this book it shares one chain, the alpha chain, with other hormones such as those that stimulate thyroid function and aspects of pregnancy and conception. The second chain, the pure beta chain, is unique to HCG. It occurs in several forms and thus three tests for it are included in the First Test Panel, two of which are done on a sample of blood serum and one on a sample of urine. This combination of tests helps to secure the result, and to reduce the risk of either a false negative or a false positive.

Many laboratories test for HCG but the limit of detection is only about 20 mIU/mL and the levels in pregnancy can go up to 300,000 mIU/mL or more. However, in testing for the Cancer Process we are interested down to levels as low as 1-2 mIU/ml. Such levels of sensitivity are only offered by very specialised laboratories. It should also be clear from this that the regular pregnancy testing kit is not adequate for testing for cancer.

Just as the presence of raised PHI is not only indicative of cancer but also presages worse to come, the same is true for increased levels of HCG. This can be anticipated, of course, since the features that it stimulates and that allow for a successful implantation of the embryo into the uterine wall and for its initial survival are also those that facilitate the development of a metastatic tumour.

HCG:

- protects the cancer cells from the activity of the host's immune system;
- increases cell proliferation;
- increases angiogenesis;
- increases the possibility of metastasis.

TK1

An enzyme called thymidine kinase (TK) catalyses part of a reaction sequence which leads to the incorporation of thymidine, one of the components of DNA, into each growing molecule of DNA. It comes in two forms: TK1 and TK2, but it is primarily TK1 that is of interest here. Initially TK1 was isolated from foetal tissue and TK2 in adult tissue and given the names foetal TK and adult TK respectively. Then it was discovered that foetal TK is associated with all rapidly-dividing cells whether in the foetus or in adults, and it was renamed TK1. The adult form is more abundant in developed tissues and is found in the mitochondria rather than in the cytoplasm. It was renamed TK2 and is independent of cell replication and not part of the First Test Panel described here.

The level of TK1 increases in foetal tissue when a cell is about to divide into two daughter cells, a process that needs the synthesis of extra DNA. Once this cell replication is complete the TK1 is broken down. This process occurs within the cell so that TK1 is not normally found in extracellular fluids, blood or other body fluids.

In adults, in normal healthy cells, TK1 is found in the cell's cytoplasm but only when cell division is about to start and undergo normal division in tissue repair or replacement. It is broken down once this replication is complete. So the level of TK1 is low in healthy people who do not have active cancer or active tissue growth and repair, such as during wound healing.

Tumour cells act differently. They use TK1 for their rapid and foetal-like DNA reproduction and cell replication, but they then release the enzyme into the circulation, probably from dead or dying tumour cells. Thus the level of TK1 can be used as a measure of malignant proliferation and give an indication of the aggressiveness of any existing tumour.

The most dramatic increases in TK1 are seen in blood cancers and it has been used to detect and monitor Non-Hodgkin's lymphoma. Several types of solid tumours have also been shown to give increased values of TK1 and the results have proven helpful in further defining the results of other tests. It is useful, for instance, in association with PSA in cases of prostate cancer. The level of PSA can be used to gain an indication of the tumour mass, whereas the level of TK1 can indicate the rate of cell proliferation. TK1 levels have been found to be increased in many solid tumours including those of the breast and kidneys and in small-cell lung cancer.

When assessing the results of this test it is important to keep the following in mind. The level of TK1 can also rise due to some non-malignant causes. These include vitamin B12 deficiency, and associated pernicious anaemia and viral infections, particularly herpes-type viruses. It can also rise during wound healing when, of course, there is increased rate of cellular replication. However, the level should return to normal within five or six weeks of surgery, or other such trauma, so if your results are high and any of these situations apply you would be wise to do a re-test at a later date.

In these last three tests, within the First Test Panel, we have, put simply:

HCG as the Autocrine Proliferating Factor, indicative of and stimulating the growth of cancer cells.

TK1 as the Autocrine Tumour Growth Factor, indicative of the rapidity of cellular reproduction.

PHI as the Autocrine Motility Factor, stimulating and facilitating metastasis.

Telomerase

Recall that when a cell multiplies it does so by dividing in half and becoming two daughter cells. To achieve this it has to double up on all the essential components in the cell so that there is one set for each daughter cell. This means that the double DNA chain of chromosomes and genes has to double. For its replication to occur correctly short elements of the chain, called telomeres, are required.

Each time the copying occurs the process does not go quite to the end of the chain but stops short one telomere before the end. This telomere is not copied and is wasted. There are a limited number of telomeres on a DNA molecule. When the DNA has been copied until there are no more telomeres left the cell can no longer divide. This is known as the Hayflick limit. While a negative consequence of this may be seen as a contribution to cell ageing and death, this process also has the benefit that it ensures that the number of replications that can occur is limited. In other words, although it induces ageing it does also inhibit the growth of excessive and unwanted tissue.

For cancer cells to keep multiplying beyond the Hayflick limit they have to find a way round this restriction. They do this by producing an enzyme, called telomerase. Telomerase catalyses the addition of more telomeres back onto the end of the DNA chain. Thus, an increase in your level of telomerase can indicate the potential of excessive cell replication and the possibility of cancer.

Telomerase is a component of the proposed First Test Panel.

An increased level of telomerase does more than indicate the probability of cancer, enabling the cells to go beyond the Hayflick limit. It also stimulates the Cancer Process in other ways, encouraging increased cancerous activity. Telomerase stimulates glycolysis, the process by which cancer cells can get energy from the cytosol by breaking down glucose. One research study has also shown that when the activity of telomerase was blocked the activity of 73 genes was reduced, including some that stimulate tumour growth, and thus tumour growth was slowed. Further, reducing the level of telomerase in cancer cells has been shown to reduce their metastatic potential.

Thus, we have the core of a panel of tests that can help to detect the earliest signs of cellular changes that are associated with cancer: HCG, PHI, lactic acid, TK1 and telomerase.

It is appropriate to consider what tests are currently available.

America Metabolic Laboratories in Florida, USA (see Appendix for details) offers, at the time of writing, a CA profile that is designed to detect the earliest signs of cancer or impending cancer. Their panel consists of three forms of HCG plus PHI, TK1 and CEA. Why three forms of HCG? HCG is a complex molecule, discussed above and this helps to improve the accuracy and reduce the risk of both false negative and false positive results. The tests for PHI and TK1 and their results are straightforward. This laboratory includes some more routine tests in their panel. They are helpful but not essential for defining cancer, however they don't increase the cost of the panel above that of costing each component individually.

CEA

The inclusion of CEA in the panel offered by American Metabolic Laboratories merits a discussion. CEA is carcino embryonic antigen. As its name implies it is active during the development of the embryo. It is a cellular adhesion protein that, like HCG, has a beneficial role to play during pregnancy, in the development of the embryo and foetus. Its activity usually stops by the time foetal development is complete and the birth occurs. Again, like HCG, its activity is counterproductive if it continues beyond this point and it can be associated with increased signs of cancer and increased risk of cancer.

It is thought that tumours that spread via the bloodstream produce or use CEA to help them adhere to healthy cells, such that they can anchor to a new location. Thus CEA encourages metastasis.

American Metabolic Laboratories does not, at the time of writing, include a test for telomerase in its CA profile, though it is thought to be working on this development. [Personal communication.] A test for telomerase is offered by Galkina Laboratory in the UK (see Appendix I).

Neither of these laboratories offers a test for lactic acid, but this can be obtained from a number of laboratories, such as Genova Diagnostics. There is a practical reason for this. Serum is the blood liquid that is left after all the cells have been removed. This is the liquid that is required for the CA profile. Serum chemistry is relatively stable and tests have shown that as long as the sample reaches the laboratory within about fourteen days of collection the test results are reliable. This would not be true for lactic acid, which should be determined on samples within 24 hours or so after the blood is collected. Samples sent to Galkina Laboratory are whole blood and do have to reach the laboratory overnight, but, again at the time of writing, they do not offer a test for lactic acid, although they have done so in the past.

Defining Cancer

It is interesting to try to define cancer, and this is an appropriate time to do so. We will leave aside, for the moment, the blood and related cancers which make up only a very small per cent of all cancers. To all intents and purposes the medical profession would seem to define cancer as the presence of a detectable tumour. Their treatment is aimed at destroying or removing this tumour. To a significant extent, they are tumour focused. If a tumour can no longer be detected you are said to be in remission. You are not said to be cured, this word is rarely used in relation to cancer. But what was happening before there was a detectable tumour?

Cancer cells are defined as ones that grow and divide more rapidly than normal, they do so in an unregulated way and they can metastasise. They can be thought of as tumour cells when they persist, increase in number and are not destroyed by other cells, such as your natural killer cells (NK cells). They are malignant when some of them are capable of separating from their origin and metastasising to another location. On this basis, cells that are producing HCG, raised levels of PHI, TK1 and CEA, and become immortal due to their production of telomerase, can be said to be cancer cells.

By the time a tumour (defined as an abnormal growth) is detectable it probably consists of millions of cells. Were they cancer cells prior to the tumour growing to a detectable size? Certainly they were. So the absence of a detectable tumour does not necessarily mean that you do not have cancer or that you are in full remission from cancer.

What about the cells that are beginning to produce HCG, TK1 and telomerase, activities common to cancer cells? Or what about those that are beginning to run short of oxygen, have slightly compromised mitochondria and electron transport chains, are beginning to turn anaerobic, and are beginning to produce increased amounts of PHI? They are not healthy cells, are they cancer cells? It is better to think of cancer as a process, a process that starts with the earliest deviation from normal or healthy cells and ends with a fully detectable tumour.

This is an important point to consider when you do the tests suggested here. It is common to hear someone say, when they get some abnormal results, "Does this mean I have cancer?" An appropriate answer could be, "You are probably somewhere along the cancer process, but possibly at a very early stage, such that a recovery programme should be relatively straightforward and further progression can be slowed, halted or even reversed."

Cure

It is rare to find people talking about a 'cure' for cancer; rightly so. Cancer is always a threat. It is a threat if you have never had cancer. It is just as much a threat if you have had cancer, one or more times, and are said to be in remission. It is not like some of the childhood diseases, such as mumps or measles, such that once you have had them, you have built up a resistance to any future repeat. If you had cancer many years ago you would be wise to resist the temptation to say that you are 'cured', which could suggest the need for no further action or care.

It is better to think of cancer as a manageable disease. You could liken it to diabetes, or to hunger or thirst. That may seem an outrageous thought, but hunger is not something you cure. You manage it. When you are hungry you eat. When you are thirsty you drink. You manage the repeat sensations. You manage diabetes by modifying your diet, reducing your intake of sugar and glucose-rich foods, by ensuring your intake of essential nutrients including vitamin B3, chromium and vanadium. Similarly you can manage cancer, either by avoiding it or by keeping it under control. This you can do by ensuring your diet and lifestyle are such as to limit your risk of either developing cancer or reactivating it. In other words, you manage cancer by following a lifestyle that helps you to avoid it.

Doing the tests in either or both of the test panels will help you to monitor your situation.

CHAPTER 12

THE SECOND TEST PANEL

If the results of the First Test Panel indicate the presence of cancer you will want to know what to do about it and how to plan your recovery programme. This is the aim of the Second Test Panel. The items tested for in this panel will give you more details as to specific aspects of your cancer and this, in turn, will indicate what you most need to focus upon to achieve a recovery.

As before, in relation to the First Test Panel, you may hear the tests described here criticised for not providing the location of a tumour, so it is worth repeating the following. These tests cover the whole body. This is not a disadvantage; it is one of their great benefits. They do not give us the location as to where the eventual tumour will occur, or perhaps has occurred, but that is not of paramount importance in this approach to the early detection of, and recovery, from cancer. In the methods proposed in this series the aim is to restore homeostasis, the normal healthy cellular function of the whole body, and to return it to a state where cancer cannot exist. There is no war or fight in this approach to cancer, no tumour to kill, or at least, not as a primary focus. There is instead a gentle effort to work harmoniously with the body and return it to normal health and function.

In general, there is an unwillingness, on the part of the medical profession, to run screening tests on a wide scale, especially those aimed at prevention rather than treatment. Prevention involves lifestyle changes and the way you shop for foods and supplements. There is no profit in this for the medical industry. Allowing cancer to develop and then subjecting the individual to medical treatments leads to many costly, patented and profitable medical procedures.

It is suggested here, that if the two test panels described and discussed in this book were made widely available, and if individuals were willing to do them and, based on the results, to make any indicated and necessary changes to their lifestyle and diet, a significant proportion of cases of cancer and of early deaths from cancer, could be avoided. This could also result in a great reduction to the overall healthcare expenditure, though also, potentially, a related reduction to the medical profit for the people involved.

Doing the tests described here and appropriately utilising the results, by modifications to lifestyle and diet, and the use of naturopathic and CAM methods to correct any abnormal results, could save your life.

In *Cancer Concerns* I discussed some of the dangers and disadvantages of both waiting for sufficient tumour mass that you could biopsy, and of having a biopsy. The results of the tests described in this book will give you much more information than you will obtain from a biopsy. They will alert you to any problem very much sooner than waiting for a detectable biopsy, they do not carry the risks that are inherent in doing one or more biopsies and they help you and your practitioner to plan your recovery programme.

The proposed Second Test Panel consists of some or all of the following:

p53 gene expression
mutated p53 gene expression
p53 protein
BAX gene expression
Bcl-2 gene expression
survivin gene expression
VEGF gene expression
MMP-2 gene expression

You may have done the First Test Panel and had some results suggesting that you are in the active Cancer Process. What do you do next? It is one thing to know that you have started along the Cancer Process; it is another to know what to do about this. When planning a recovery programme it is important to know what you are facing and how best to get a positive result from whatever you plan to do.

The tests in the proposed Second Test Panel can help in this. Most of these tests are offered by Galkina Laboratory in Bournemouth, UK, but they may also be available elsewhere. However, you should aim to find a practitioner experienced in this field rather than contacting the laboratory directly, and you will certainly need a practitioner's referral before the tests can be done or any results sent out to you. This office is happy to assist if such help is required.

The tests in this panel will define aspects of cancer that need attention and provide the information on which a recovery plan can be built.

Once you have the results you will want to take action to correct any that are out of the normal range. This is a highly complex process and will be described in the next book in this series, entitled *Targeting Cancer*. It is beyond the scope of this book, and you should work with a practitioner that can advise and assist you, probably the one that helped you to organise the tests. The point of the discussion here is:

(a) to alert you to the possibilities that are open to you;
(b) to give you a tool to help you choose your practitioner;
(c) to help your practitioner in guiding you towards recovery.

Genes, Proteins and Enzymes

The following tests relate to genes and the activity of the proteins for which they code. You may find that your level of the gene expression has been determined or the level of the protein itself. You may find that the discussion uses the terms protein, protease or enzyme somewhat interchangeably. Understanding these interconnections will help you to understand what is being discussed. The actual amount of each gene is small, but this can be misleading and may lead you to underestimate them. If the product is an enzyme or catalyst, these enzymes can catalyse many thousands of repeats of the same reaction in less than a second, thus the effect of even a small amount of an unwanted enzyme, or an inadequate supply of a desirable enzyme, can be very large indeed.

Protein 53

A protein called protein 53 or p53 has been called the 'guardian of the threshold'. It is one of the most important compounds in relation to your protection from cancer. It was discovered in 1979 and is now known to perform several valuable functions. It is a tumour suppressor gene, one that hinders the production of cancer cells, and was the first one to be discovered. It sits inside the nucleus of each cell and makes sure the DNA doubling that is required, when a cell is dividing into two daughter cells, is done correctly.

If a fault or mutation occurs during the process of doubling the amount of DNA and this fault is found in one or both of the DNA strands in the daughter cells, p53 is activated. It targets genes that initiate actions aimed at repairing the damaged or mutated DNA. If that repair fails, p53 sends out signals that causes apoptosis and so leads to the death of these faulty daughter cells. The increased output of p53 also triggers the production of another protective protein, p21. Further, p53 regulates the electron transport chain, the sequence of reactions whose early damage is an initiating factor in the development of cancer. It does even more and inhibits angiogenesis, the building of new blood vessels that would be needed by any tumour that formed and tried to nourish itself and grow. p53 stimulates the production of BAX (see below) that in turn stimulates apoptosis. From this it is clear that p53 is a very valuable protective agent in regard to preventing both the start and the continuance of cancer.

In summary, p53:

* detects faulty DNA replication;
* endeavours to correct these faults;
* triggers apoptosis if this correction fails;
* stimulates the production of protective p21;
* regulates the electron transport chain;
* stimulates BAX and inhibits Bcl-2 (see below) so increases apoptosis, when that is called for;
* inhibits excessive angiogenesis;
* inhibits survivin (see below).

Three of the tests in the Second Test Panel relate to this protein. The level of the gene that triggers the synthesis of the protein can be determined, as can the level of the protein itself. In addition, the presence of the mutated or damaged form of the protein can be ascertained. Ideally all three should be tested.

In cancer-free health the level of p53 is generally low. There is just sufficient present to ensure that DNA replications are proceeding correctly. If the levels of the gene and the protein are above normal it suggests the existence of cancer but does also suggest that the cells are fighting the cancer. If cancer has been diagnosed and the level of the p53 gene or protein has not risen, this suggests that there is insufficient anti-cancer activity. The situation is even worse if the p53 gene itself is mutated. If that happens the mutated form can build up in the nucleus. Because it is mutated it fails to do the job of p53. Further, it inhibits any p53 that is present and reduces its effectiveness. This mutation is one that is commonly found in the blood of people with cancer and needs to be corrected.

BAX and Bcl-2

In health, apoptosis, or self-regulated cell suicide, occurs in any cell that is faulty. A number of compounds encourage or stimulate apoptosis and others inhibit apoptosis. The combination of these two groups provides an appropriate system of checks and balances. If you have cancer and they are out of their correct balance, this can worsen the situation.

BAX and Bcl-2 are two of a group of compounds that impact apoptosis. These two work in opposition to each other. BAX stimulates apoptosis and should be fully active to help destroy faulty cells and so to both prevent and fight cancer. Its activity is triggered by p53.

Bcl-2 is an anti-apoptotic protein. Its action allows faulty and cancerous cells to survive and multiply. Bcl-2 is hindered by increased levels of p53, yet another way in which p53 is helpful. Raised levels of Bcl-2 are common in people with cancer and indicate poor response to treatment and a poor outcome. Any recovery programme should aim to stimulate BAX production and minimise the production of Bcl-2 if either of them are outside normal levels.

Survivin

Survivin is another protein that inhibits apoptosis. It has a valuable role to play in fast growing tissues and in the development of the embryo, where it is important and encourages the rapid tissue growth required by the developing embryo. However, it is rarely found associated with healthy tissue or with fully-developed and differentiated cells, but is common in the blood of people with cancer. There are at least three problems when increased levels of survivin are found in the blood:

- When it is present it suggests that the cancer is present and particularly aggressive.
- It stimulates and encourages cancer.
- It inhibits or blocks the action of many therapeutic agents, be they natural compounds or chemotherapy agents or other drugs.

Protein 53 is active again here in that it helps to reduce the level of survivin. There are also several natural remedies that can do this.

Vascular Endothelial Growth Factor (VEGF)

Any growing tissue needs its own increased supply of blood and this is achieved by a process known as angiogenesis. Increased angiogenesis leads to several outcomes:

- It allows nutrients to reach the newly developing cells;
- It allows for the removal of waste products of cellular metabolism; and
- It allows the cell to receive information and instructions from the rest of your body and to communicate with the tissues elsewhere in your body.

Angiogenesis is needed by growing tissues during growth and in tissue repair and wound healing. In these situations angiogenesis is needed and is beneficial. However, a developing tumour also needs its own supply of blood, and when angiogenesis is stimulated for this purpose it is harmful to the individual.

Many compounds are called into play when new blood vessels are growing. They stimulate and assist the process. One of these is Vascular Endothelial Growth Factor, or VEGF, and a test for this is a component of the proposed Second Test Panel.

Angiogenesis is yet another example of a process that, under the correct circumstances, is important and valuable, even essential, but that, in relation to cancer it is undesirable. It is a beneficial process, gone wrong.

Matrix Metalloproteinases (MMPases)

Six features that have been labelled 'the hallmarks of cancer', are common to cancer cells, and are an essential part of their development and survival. These include:

- self-sufficiency in growth signals;
- insensitivity to growth-inhibiting signals;
- avoidance of apoptosis;
- limitless replication potential;
- on-going angiogenesis; and
- metastatic potential.[38, 39]

Of these, the first five apply to benign tumours as well as to malignant tumours. In effect, they have already been considered by the previous tests. Benign tumours may grow; they may resist apoptosis and encourage angiogenesis. They are space occupying and may cause harm by blocking essential processes or damaging the local tissue in some way, but they are rarely fatal. What makes cancer so dangerous is its ability to spread to and invade other tissues, to metastasise. It is the metastatic potential or capability that is an essential feature of malignant cancer development.

The process of metastasis is not nearly as simple or as easy as many people seem to imagine. There are many important and difficult steps that need to be taken. Many compounds are called into play to enable the initial tumour to release cells, for these cells to break into the bloodstream, then break out of the bloodstream across the blood vessel wall, invade the new tissue and establish a metastatic location.

An important step in this process is the weakening of the target tissue such that the migrating cells can penetrate it. One of the most active groups of such compounds is the group of matrix metalloproteinase (MMPase) enzymes. There are several of them but a particularly important one, and one that is included in this Second Test Panel is MMP-2ase. The level of this is commonly raised in cancer. This too can be detected in the blood.

Summary

It is noteworthy that many of the compounds, reactions and strategies that encourage cancer are also those that are active during foetal growth, when rapid growth and development is desirable, and when tissue repair is needed. Thus, the Cancer Process is not something entirely new to the body. It is made up of processes that had their time and place during foetal development, but that, in health, will largely have ceased to function. Once cancer is triggered they have become reactivated, inappropriately, by carcinogens and lifestyle errors. These have triggered the mitochondrial failure and altered cellular chemistry and gene expression as discussed above.

That, in brief, is what is discussed in much greater detail and more depth in the thesis that comprises Section II and which follows. If you are familiar with this material, in Section I, it should help you if you choose to explore Section II in more detail. Although much of Section II is very technical, some of it is descriptive and readily understood. These sections include the concepts described by Pasteur and Béchamp, and the case histories towards the end of Section II.

Even if you only skim over the more technical aspects of Section II and pick up on the segments that appeal to you, this can help you to increase your understanding and knowledge. It will help you to realise the extent of the solid science, the research and the biochemical underpinning of what is being recommended here. This can help you to feel more confident in the benefit of the tests and in greater control of the processes and changes in your life that are inevitably being encouraged by your CAM practitioner. It may also help you when you want to refute, either to yourself or others, the often-made claim that alternative or CAM procedures are based on unproven or unsound ideas.

It should be clear by now that there is an immense amount of proven, evidence-based, and soundly biochemically-based research and knowledge behind both these tests and the use of an alternative approach to the management of cancer.

If you decide to give this book to your practitioner and ask them to organise the tests for you, at least if you have read Section I, here, you will have a better understanding of what your results mean when you are given them.

You can use the information in Section II if you come up against people, be they friends and relatives or parts of your medical team, who try to insist that there is no sound, proven test-basis for the alternative options you may want to follow. You can show this to your doctor, for instance, if you want to enlist his/her support.

The good news is that there are natural remedies, mostly nutrients and a variety of plants (herbs or foods) that can help to correct any of the imbalances that are found by these tests. Again, this is a job for your professional healthcare practitioner. It is also the subject matter of the next book in this series, *Targeting Cancer*.

Second Test Panel

Core tests: Protein 53 (gene, wild protein and mutated protein), BAX, Bcl-2, survivin, VEGF, MMP-2

Optional: Protein 21, p185

CHAPTER 13

DOING THE TESTS

The Decision

Many people tell me they would not like to do these tests, or that they are too afraid to do them, because the disease is so awful and the treatment is so horrific they couldn't face it. They would prefer not to know, to stick their head in the sand and hope it wasn't going to happen to them.

But consider this. These tests will detect the very earliest signs and stages of the Cancer Process. They can detect the cellular changes long before a doctor is interested in them or willing to pay any attention to them, and certainly long before they will advise any of their medical treatment options. So even if the results indicate the start of the Cancer Process you will not be faced with any hard decisions or any heavy persuasion from family and friends, to leap into some of the toxic and unpleasant medical treatments.

The corrections and aids to recovery, or the normal restoration of homeostasis and general return to total health, at this early stage, are simple and straightforward. They involve improving your diet, and thus in all likelihood improving your general health as well as reversing the Cancer Process. They involve avoiding toxins and improving your lifestyle, which could lead to improving your level of energy and your sense of wellbeing. They probably involve taking supplements, nutrients or plant-based compounds, that will, at the very least, help you to avoid other health issues, now and in the future, and will also help to reverse the Cancer Process.

There is another aspect to this. You may well have had concerns about cancer, wondering whether or not you have it or are developing it. These concerns could be small ones, niggling ones, pushed to the back of your mind. They could be larger and causing you even greater concern. If you do these tests, particularly the First Test Panel, and the results are all normal, it can give you some assurance that, at least for now, all is well. I say 'for now' as cancer is an on-going threat to everyone. It is estimated that it is either our most common cause of death or is becoming so. Statistics can give many and different answers. Much depends on the words actually written on the death certificate. Was it cancer or was it pneumonia that was the actual cause of death, if the person had both? Doing the First Test Panel, perhaps annually or biannually, can give you on-going reassurance. All being well, it can put your mind at rest and your worries behind you.

If you do have cancer, doing the Second Test Panel will help you and your practitioner to provide a more targeted approach to designing your recovery programme. Repeated use of the Second Test Panel will help you to monitor your progress and make any modifications to your programme that are required. Then, when these results are normal, doing the First Test Panel will help you to make sure that all traces of cancer have been removed.

Another reason to do the proposed First Test Panel concerns the situation if you have already had a cancer diagnosis, followed by treatment and been told that 'they got it all', or that there is no longer any sign of cancer and that you are in remission. The same considerations apply here. The results of the First Test Panel will give you, if normal, even greater assurance that they did get it all and that all is well. Alternatively, if the results are abnormal, they will warn you that they did not, at the cellular level, 'get it all' and that you have more to do to capitalise on whatever treatment you have been through and to avoid a fully-developed recurrence and having to do it again.

You almost certainly do regular services on your car, but if you don't and if it fails, at least it can be replaced. You are irreplaceable. Regularly servicing is important.

Practical Details

As described here, there are two proposed test panels. In fact, at the time of writing, they do not exist as specific offerings by any one specific laboratory. However approximations do exist.

First Test Panel	Second Test Panel	CA Profile by American Metabolic Laboratories (USA)	Galkina Laboratory (UK)
HCG (IMM)		HCG (IMM)	
HCG (IRMA)		HCG (IRMA)	
HCG (urine)		HCG (urine)	
PHI		PHI	
CEA		CEA	
TK1		TK1	
Telomerase		In development	Telomerase
TM2-PK (optional)			TM2-PK
Lactic acid (other laboratories)			
	p53, gene, mutated and protein		p53, gene, mutated and protein
	p21 (optional)		p21
	p185 (optional)		p185
	BAX		BAX
	Bcl-2		Bcl-2
	survivin		survivin
	VEGF		VEGF
	MMP-2		MMP-2
		Optional other tests. Discuss with your practitioner.	Many other useful tests.

Sample Collection

The CA profile offered by American Metabolic Laboratories utilises two samples. One of these is an early morning urine sample. This can be collected by the individual and placed in the small sample tube provided in the kit supplied by the laboratory and given to you by your practitioner. The other is a serum sample. To collect this you need to visit a phlebotomy laboratory (one that draws a vial of blood and can then process the sample). At the phlebotomy centre a vial of blood will be drawn from one of your veins. This then has to be allowed to stand for twenty minutes so that clot formation starts. It is then centrifuged, or spun, so that all the blood cells fall or are thrown to the bottom of the tube. This is essential as the presence of any blood cells in the sample that is sent for analysis will lead to faulty and misleading results. The clear liquid (serum) can then be drawn off the top and placed in the second small tube that is part of the sample kit.

These two samples are then posted to the laboratory in Florida, USA. Because there are no cells involved, or the sample is not 'live', time is not critical. The laboratory's studies have shown that the sample is essentially stable for up to two weeks, although it is presumably better to have it reach the laboratory sooner rather than later. This does mean that a good regular postal service, or one that promises a slightly greater speed of delivery, is usually adequate. As a result, samples sent from outside the USA can be readily dealt with. The laboratory usually charges the practitioner for the test panel and they in turn will generally charge the individual. Results are usually obtained within two to nine days of receipt of the sample by the laboratory. Results are sent by email. Hard copies can also be obtained. The details and their significance can then be discussed with your practitioner.

The procedure is somewhat different for the Second Test Panel. Live blood is used and should arrive at the laboratory within 24 to 48 hours of collection, or as soon as possible. If in doubt this should be discussed with the laboratory beforehand. There is sufficient margin in this schedule for samples to be delivered to the laboratory from anywhere in the world, but it also means that they will have to be sent by a fast courier service if they are sent from outside the UK. Inside the UK they can be sent by First Class post. They should be sent between Monday and Wednesday so that they arrive on Thursday or Friday and can be stabilised immediately and not left to stand until after the weekend.

There are two methods of collecting the blood samples for the tests in this Second Test Panel. Firstly, a vial of venous blood can be collected at a phlebotomy laboratory in the usual way, via a needle into a vein. If this method is used, the Galkina laboratory requires a referral from a medical doctor before they will do the analysis and they will only send the results back to that doctor. It is up to the patient to obtain the results from their chosen doctor or to ensure that the results are sent on to any naturopath or alternative practitioner with whom they are working.

In the second method, a sample of capillary blood can be collected. This can be done by any practitioner, medical or naturopathic. A finger prick is required and enough blood is squeezed out to fill a very small tube. The laboratory does not then require a medical referral and will accept a referral from a naturopath or other CAM practitioner. They will also return the results to the referring naturopath. Such are the vagaries of the UK law, current at the time of writing.

Payment for this panel of tests has to accompany the sample to the laboratory. The results are usually obtained within three weeks. You should then consult with your practitioner as to their significance and the uses that can be made of them when planning your recovery protocol.

Laboratories

American Metabolic Laboratories,
Director: Dr E. Schandl
Address: 1818 Sheriden Street, Suite 102, Hollywood, Florida FL 33020, USA
www.caprofile.net
Email: info@caprofile.net
T: 1-954-929-4814
Tests: HCG, PHI, CEA, TK1, (telomerase, in development)

The Galkina Laboratory Limited
Director: Dr O. Galkina
Address: 681 Wimbourne Road, Bournemouth, Dorset, BH9 2AT, UK
www.neuro-lab.com
Email: drtaylor@thegalkinalab.co.uk
T: 44-1202-510910

The second panel of tests consists of: p53 gene and p53 protein mutated and wild, p21 (optional), BAX, Bcl-2, MMP-2, survivin, and VEGF. This laboratory also offers tests for telomerase that are suggested as part of the First Test Panel. It offers many other tests including detailed testing of immune factors and neurotransmitters.

Genova Diagnostics
Address: 63 Zillicoa Street, Asheville, NC 28801, USA
www.gdx.net
Email via website
T: 800-522-4762: 1-828-253-0621

Tests: The Optimum Nutritional Evaluation (ONE) test and a test for lactic acid, plus many other general but useful tests.

Other Laboratories

If any other laboratories are offering all or some of these tests this author would be delighted to hear from them and to include the information in future editions of this book. They can also be added to the author's website: www.xandriawilliams.co.uk

SECTION II

A thesis submitted in part fulfilment of the requirements for
the
**Degree of Doctor of Philosophy in Natural Health
Science**
at the University of Natural Medicine
Santa Fe, New Mexico, USA, 2012

THE VERY EARLY DETECTION OF CANCER

TWO PROPOSED TEST PANELS FOR THE VERY EARLY DETECTION OF CANCER AND PLANNING A RECOVERY PROGRAMME

By

Xandria Williams

ABSTRACT

Cancer is a process, the end result of which is a tumour. Cancer is not defined by the presence or absence of a tumour, but by the absence of any signs that this Cancer Process is operative. It is a process of cellular changes that occur in cells throughout the body.

Cancer is almost entirely (arguably 93% or more) a disease of diet and lifestyle, in the broadest sense, and so cancer is a readily preventable disease for those willing to make appropriate changes to their diet and lifestyle. If present, it can be corrected by complementary, alternative and metabolic (CAM) therapies that correct the observed errors by supportive and non-toxic means. These corrections will be most effective when started as close as possible to the start of the Cancer Process. In this thesis two panels of tests are proposed. They can be used concurrently or sequentially, in their entirety or piecemeal, as symptoms and other clinical indications dictate, and can detect the Cancer Process within weeks of its initiation.

The use of panels of tests, rather than single tests, improves the detection rate and minimises the possibility of false negative results. By proposing remedial actions based on non-toxic, health promoting lifestyle changes, false positive results to the test are, although important, a lesser concern than false negative results, provided a full explanation of the implications are given to the individual and only CAM, and not toxic MDS (medical drug surgery), therapies are introduced at this time. The focus of the First Test Panel is to detect the start of the Cancer Process. Evidence is given for the effectiveness of a First Test Panel consisting of human chorionic gonadotropin (HCG), phosphohexose isomerase (PHI), carcino embryonic antigen (CEA), telomerase and lactic acid. A major focus of this thesis is on the prevalence of HCG in a wide variety of cancers.

Further corroborative tests are proposed out of which a Second Test Panel can be selected. They include p53 protein, gene, mutated and wild, p21 protein, p185 protein, and the genes that code for BAX, Bcl-2, matrix metalloproteinase-2 (MMP-2), vascular endothelial growth factor (VEGF) and survivin. These tests serve to confirm or deny and elaborate the results of the First Test Panel, and can provide information as to the most appropriate components of a recovery programme.

Cancer is fast becoming the major health concern and killer in the Western world. Such tests are relatively inexpensive and readily available. If the results are acted upon, they could make a significant positive impact on overall health improvement and the cost of healthcare.

Currently, the dominant paradigm in medical practice is that cancer is the result of genetic aberrations and commences with, or is defined by, the presence of a tumour. The approach argued for in this thesis, that it results from lifestyle-induced cellular changes at the mitochondrial level, conflicts with this paradigm but leads to a targeted and constructive preventative and therapeutic approach.

Case histories are given as examples of the use of these two test panels.

PROPOSITION

Cancer is a process of progressive and systemic cellular failure leading to a tumour as a final end product. The cellular changes are essentially due to diet and lifestyle errors in the broadest sense. Even the small percentage of cancers for which a genetic predisposition is claimed can be affected, positively or negatively, by these errors. A significant improvement can be achieved by correcting or removing the causative factors and correcting the metabolic errors. The closer to the start of the Cancer Process that this intervention is initiated the greater is the likelihood of success.

This early detection should not be delayed until a tumour is detected. It is of paramount importance that a chemical test, or panel of tests, such as is presented here, of blood, urine or other body fluids, be established and provide the earliest possible detection. It is proposed here that such a First Test Panel consists of analysing HCG, PHI, CEA, lactic acid and telomerase.

It is further proposed that a Second Test Panel, once the Cancer Process has been identified or seems likely in an individual, should consist of a minimum of p53, BAX, Bcl-2, MMP-2, survivin and VEGF; other tests can be included as required. This Second Test Panel can further secure the diagnosis. It can provide indications of the cellular and physiological corrections that need to be made to diet and lifestyle and point to the natural remedies that are required. All of the therapeutic interventions can be achieved by natural, non-toxic means. Once the fear of the treatment is removed, individuals are more likely to be willing to undertake the First Test Panel and focus on prevention or early discovery and early treatment intervention.

The test selections are based on an understanding of the underlying biochemistry and physiology and the metabolic errors that lead to the Cancer Process, plus extensive searches into the research results of other clinicians. This is followed by the clinical experience of their application and their usefulness in planning a recovery programme.

INTRODUCTION

People today who are concerned about the prevention, diagnosis or treatment of cancer are faced with a dilemma. Should they follow the medical, drug, surgery (MDS) route or the complementary, alternative, metabolic (CAM) route, or should they hedge their bets and combine the two?

A diminishing majority of people take it for granted that following the MDS route is, although often highly unpleasant and rarely fully successful, the best, most sure and evidence-based approach to take and that the CAM route is based on 'unproven' methods. This is not so. As this thesis will help to show, the CAM route, correctly utilised, is every bit as sure and evidence-based as the MDS route, arguably even more so. There is an enormous amount of biochemical, physiological and clinical research written up in peer-reviewed, PubMed, academic journals and related sources, that attests to both the benefits of, and the lack of harm to be derived from, the CAM options.

When comparing the two approaches a brief look at recent history is helpful. It concerns two Frenchman of the 19th century, Louis Pasteur and Antoine Béchamp who viewed health, the activities of microorganisms, and the development of disease, from diametrically opposite perspectives.

In the middle of the 19th century Louis Pasteur identified and publicised information about the presence of bacteria and other pathogens at the site of infections. He then made the mental leap required to claim that the pathogen had caused the infection. Antoine Béchamp, also French and of a similar age, observed the same phenomenon but took the reverse view. He considered it was the breakdown of the terrain, the person's weakened or previously damaged tissues, that caused the disease and that the pathogens arrived later and were opportunistic beneficiaries rather than causative agents. Béchamp stated that this explained why one person succumbed to a particular health problem while another, in the same location or situation, did not. The two men had many debates during the course of their professional lives, but it is Pasteur who, at the end of his life, changed his mind and acknowledged, 'It's the terrain that is important'.

Unfortunately, the initial ideas of Pasteur were seized upon by the many drug companies of the day and this continues to the present. It is easy to focus on finding drugs that are patentable and profitable and that will kill specific microorganisms. Whether or not that ensures long-term health is debatable. On the other hand, it is impossible to make and patent profitable ways of improving the individual's terrain, for this depends on good diet, a healthy lifestyle, the avoidance of toxins and, if necessary, the use of nutrients, herbs, specific phytonutrient-rich foods and natural remedies, none of which can be patented. Thus, the ideas of Béchamp were largely ignored, even though, in the end, Pasteur came round to them and embraced them.

This thinking informs the medical profession and the MDS system to this day with regard to much of medicine in relation to cancer. Pasteur's approach leads to the present focus on attacking, removing or destroying the tumour which is seen, largely, as the cause of the problem. Béchamp's approach, of improving the terrain, the overall health of the body, restoring homeostasis and appreciating the body's ability to cure itself, provided it is given all the nutrients and related substances that it needs, and is not subjected to the toxins of the day, leads to the CAM approach.

On this basis it is worth tabulating the differences between the MDS and the CAM approach to cancer.

	CAM	MDS
Cancer	A process of changes from healthy to unhealthy cells that can be tested for and changed.	The presence of a tumour or, in relation to blood and related cancers, the detection of such major changes.
Development	Starts with small changes in cellular chemistry.	Such early changes are rarely sought or tested for.

Diagnosis	Tests for early chemical changes as discussed in this thesis.	Delayed, with few exceptions, until a tumour is found.
Confirmation	The tests offered in this thesis.	Biopsy, with risk of metastasis.
Treatment aim	Restoration of homeostasis, of normal healthy tissue and function.	Elimination of the tumour.
Treatment methods	Non-toxic, health-promoting diet and lifestyle changes plus appropriate non-toxic remedies, as indicated by the test results.	Surgery (traumatic, with general risks and risk of metastasis), chemical drugs (toxic) and radiation (can cause cancer).
Toxic effects	None.	High, from chemotherapy and radiation, some from surgery.
Remission	Confirmed when all early cellular diagnostic tests return to normal.	Assumed if a tumour can no longer be detected.

With the CAM approach as a starting point, the primary aim of this thesis has been to put forward the evidence for a panel of tests that will detect the first signs of chemical changes that can lead to cancer, and to detect these changes long before a tumour has developed. This is followed by a further group of tests from which a Second Test Panel can be selected with the aim of helping to confirm, or not, the results of the First Test Panel and to indicate positive recovery options. The two panels can be done either consecutively or concurrently, depending on the circumstances. There are several options:

* If cancer is uncertain, but a possibility, the First Test Panel can be done to determine whether or not cancer is present. If it is not, then sensible preventive lifestyle changes may be all that is required.

* If, by the results obtained, it seems likely that the Cancer Process is well established then it is recommended that the Second Test Panel be done to help construct a recovery programme.

* If a diagnosis of cancer has already been received then the Second Test Panel will again help to construct an appropriate recovery programme.

* Doing the First Test Panel at the same time will provide a base line to which the individual should aim to return on recovery. It will have a small and minor effect on planning the recovery programme.

PART I

CANCER FUNDAMENTALS

Cancer – One Disease or Many?

One school of thought has it that each location of cancer equates to a different type of cancer. This is particularly common in the MDS system where cancer is seen as a tumour and its location as one of its prime characteristics, in combination with genetic changes that are observed. The other school of thought, favoured by most CAM practitioners and the view of this author, is that cancer is a process, one that is initiated and takes place at the cellular level. It is focused on the mitochondria, in large part, regardless of the final location of a tumour once the latter forms.

It is noteworthy that, unlike other health problems, cancer is not specifically a disease or disorder of the organ or tissue in which a tumour is finally established, although ultimately the tissue in which the tumour develops may become compromised. Cancer of the lungs, for instance, is not, initially, a product of the failure of the lungs to exchange oxygen, although this may, in time, result from the presence of the tumour(s) in that location. As such, lung cancers are not treated, primarily, with medications, herbs or other natural remedies that improve lung function. Cancer of the breast is not a failure of the breast to produce milk and treated accordingly. Cancer of the ovaries is not a failure of the ovaries to perform their normal function and treated with remedies that stimulate ovulation. Cancer of the liver is not due to the liver's failure to perform all the many thousands of reactions of the liver, and it is not treated with remedies that stimulate liver function, except in so far as this helps the liver to deal with the cancer wherever it is located. When specific organs or tissues do fail, when cancer is present, it is normally the result of the presence of a space-occupying and invasive tumour that is interfering with the normal function of that tissue or organ, not primarily a failure inherent to the tissue or organ itself.

From this it can be argued that cancer is fundamentally one disease and that it locates in tissues or organs that are the most vulnerable in the individual concerned. Working from this basis a case can be made for looking for tests that will detect the earliest steps in this universal Cancer Process. Determining the ultimate location of a tumour is the second step, not the first.

Cancer as a Process

Cancer should be regarded as a process rather than be defined by the presence of a tumour. This process involves the whole body. It starts with cellular changes that can be detected and monitored months and probably years before a tumour forms, possibly in as few as six weeks after they start. These changes start, or are first expressed, in the mitochondria by a faulty electron transport chain and compromised oxidative phosphorylation. Testing for these changes or the resultant presence of unwanted chemical compounds should be a vital part of prevention and early detection programmes. This discussion focuses on solid tumours, although the application of the results can be applied to almost all cancers.

Cancer is an immensely challenging disease once it has been detected, usually in the form of a tumour or blood changes. Prevention is, as always, very much more effective than cure. Failing prevention, the earliest possible detection is highly desirable. Once a tumour is detected it is possible that it has been developing for many months, even years. Recent research[40] suggests that cancer cells may spread around the body much earlier than was previously thought.[41]

There is growing evidence that by the time a tumour has been detected, cancer cells may already have spread to other sites. This being the case, the emphasis for a sudden rush to surgery is reduced. It is now thought possible that healthy cells can carry cancer cells to new sites where they can lie dormant until the key genes are activated and stimulate these cells into reproduction and growth.[42] These findings help to explain why some metastatic tumours can develop long after the original tumour has been removed or been destroyed by radiation or other means. This is true even if a wide margin of clear or healthy tissue surrounding the tumour has been removed. Discovery at this late date is too late for truly early intervention or prevention of recurrence.

It is imperative that non-invasive, simple and economic tests be found and utilised; tests that can detect early biochemical changes anywhere in the body. Ideally such tests should not be invasive, nor should they cause potential harm to the body in any way, such as can occur as a result of mammograms, PAP smears or biopsies. Such tests should also relate to the whole body. There should be no need to test every organ or type of tissue, possibly by a variety of tests each time. In this holistic way the result(s) can give information that is far more comprehensive than single tissue or organ tests such as those PAP smears, PSA results or mammograms.

In a medical system where cancer is defined, largely, by the presence or absence of a tumour and where treatment is focused almost entirely on eradicating or destroying the tumour, the first requirement is limited to knowing the location of the tumour. As such, little attention is paid, by conventional medical practitioners, to systemic or pre-tumour cancerous changes. The tests suggested here come into the realm of prevention and this is rarely practised within conventional medicine. In fact, modern medicine is unlikely to embrace or use these tests as its practitioners will almost certainly not have, or be allowed to use, the tools needed to help the individual make the appropriate corrections to any errors that are found among the results. Metabolic errors and early cellular changes cannot be corrected by any of their three methods, by surgery, chemotherapy or radiation.

In a system of health that focuses on the health, function and wellbeing of the whole body and, where necessary, correcting any errors that are found, the focus is less on the need to know the location of the tumour and more on detecting and correcting these very early errors as rapidly as possible. In this system the focus of therapy will be on improving the state of the whole body, from the cellular level upwards. Nonetheless, if a tumour is located, any treatment programme may well include modifications relevant to the location and type of the tumour(s).

Very Early Warning Signs

Cancer is, arguably, a readily preventable disease. This being so, any early warning sign that might indicate an increased risk of developing cancer should be watched for, noted and acted upon. This segment covers suggestions as to just a few of these very early indications. They can occur even before the first cancer cells form and so can come into play before the use of either of the two test panels that are the subject of this thesis. They are not discussed in detail here, but the concept deserves mention, however briefly.

Common Risk Factors for cancer are well known to include smoking, obesity, excessive alcohol consumption, ionising radiation, toxins and pollution, infections, hyperglycaemia, physical inactivity, and finally, stress, particularly of the type where the individual feels helpless and hopeless about things they feel they cannot change. It has been proposed by many that a common link between these factors and cancer is inflammation, and early signs of inflammation can be tested for and could provide warnings, even before the test panels, proposed here, come into play.

As evidence for the link between inflammation and cancer Anand et al[43] cite the following:

* Inflammatory markers that have been closely linked with tumourigenesis include:

    cytokines (TNF, IL-1, IL-6, and chemokines);

    enzymes (COX-2, 5-LOX, and matrix metalloproteinase-9 [MMP-9]);

    adhesion molecules (such as intercellular adhesion molecule, endothelium leukocyte adhesion molecule 1, and vascular cell adhesion molecule 1).
* All of these inflammatory gene products are regulated by nuclear transcription factor, NF-κB.
* Most chemotherapeutic agents and γ-radiation, used for the treatment of cancers, lead to activation of NF-κB.
* NF-κB controls the expression of other gene products linked with tumourigenesis such as tumour antiapoptotics (Bcl-2, Bcl-xL, IAP-1, IAP-2, XIAP, survivin, cFLIP, and TRAF-1), proliferation factors (such as c-myc and cyclin D1), invasion facilitators (MMP-9), and angiogenesis stimulators (vascular endothelial growth factor [VEGF]).
* In most cancers, chronic inflammation precedes tumourigenesis.

* Most carcinogens and other risk factors (above) have been shown to activate NF-κB.

* Constitutive NF-κB activation has been encountered in most types of cancers.

* Activation of NF-κB has been linked with chemoresistance and radioresistance.

* Suppression of NF-κB inhibits the proliferation of tumours, leads to apoptosis, inhibits invasion, and suppresses angiogenesis.

* Polymorphisms of TNF, IL-1, IL-6, and cyclin D1 genes encountered in various cancers are all regulated by NF-κB, and mutations in genes encoding for inhibitors of NF-κB have been found in certain cancers.

* Almost all chemopreventive agents described above suppress NF-κB activation.

The following tests are just a few examples of ways to detect inflammation and could provide some early warning clues as to whether or not the individual is heading towards an active Cancer Process. They are tests that may have been done for some other health reason and, if the results are outside the normal range, they should not be ignored, in relation to cancer as well as for whatever other reason the tests were done.

C-reactive protein (CRP)

Protein is commonly released at inflammatory sites and can be detected in a blood sample. One of the most common is C-reactive protein (CRP) which is synthesised in the liver, stimulated by interleukin-6 (IL-6). It is generally a more reliable marker of inflammation than the erythrocyte sedimentation rate (ESR). Persistent high levels of CRP are known not only to indicate inflammation but also to persist when cancer develops, and to suggest a poor prognosis, both in relation to any types of inflammation and specifically in relation to cancer.[44, 45, 46, 47]

Tumour Necrosis Factor (TNF)

TNF is produced by a wide range of cells including several of the immune system, and is an integral part of the inflammatory process. It promotes apoptosis and causes necrosis in some forms of cancer but stimulates growth of other types. Overall high levels have been correlated with poor survival prognosis.[48]

Interleukin-6 (IL-6)

IL-6 plays a variety of roles in relation to inflammation and cancer, being both pro- and anti-inflammatory. In prostate cancer, for instance, it has been shown to change its function from that of a paracrine growth inhibitor to that of an autocrine growth stimulator.[49] Raised levels are known to occur in inflammation and in cancer. They have shown a reduced survival time in lung cancer.[50] St John et al[51] have shown that both IL-6 in serum and Interleukin-8 (IL-8) in saliva are good biomarkers for oral cavity and oropharyngeal cancer. In addition, IL-8, also associated with inflammation, is known to promote angiogenesis and metastasis.[52]

There are many other markers of inflammation, from tests that might be done for a variety of reasons. If they do show indications of active inflammation, or if there are clinical symptoms of ongoing inflammation, these should encourage improvement in diet and lifestyle and an increased focus on cancer prevention.

Tests

In this thesis several such compounds, and the tests for them, are discussed with these concepts in mind. The tests can be considered to make up two panels. The initial panel focuses on whether or not the individual has started along the Cancer Process. The Second Test Panel serves to confirm the diagnosis from the first and to provide more detailed information as to the appropriate goals of any treatment plan.

FIRST TEST PANEL

The compounds in the First Test Panel include Human Chorionic Gonadotropin (HCG), Phospho Hexose Isomerase (PHI), Carcino Embryonic Antigen (CEA), Tumour Marker-2 Pyruvate Kinase (TM2-PK), lactic acid and telomerase. All of these compounds, individually, offer valuable prognostic information in relation to both the early detection of cancer and the monitoring of the Cancer Process and the results of therapeutic interventions. Collectively they can offer an even more informative picture and a more secure diagnosis.

Human Chorionic Gonadotropin (HCG) is a hormone produced by placental cells and used to detect the start, or stage, of pregnancy. In relation to cancer it is generally thought by most clinical doctors and oncologists, to be produced by and only significant for the detection of cancers related to pregnancy or the gonads. In this thesis it will be shown that it is now known to be produced by almost one hundred different types of cancers, a number which may well rise as the research continues. Further, the most sensitive tests now available are able to detect low levels of HCG at about the sixth week after the formation of the first cancer cells. HCG and its detection in serum or urine is thus a highly valuable early marker for the start of the Cancer Process. Testing for HCG has many advantages over taking and analysing a biopsy sample. This is discussed below.

Phospho Hexose Isomerase (PHI) is a critical enzyme in the cytosol's Embden-Meyerhof (E-M) pathway that describes the anaerobic conversion of six-carbon glucose to three-carbon pyruvic acid. This pathway is also referred to as glycolysis, although the latter term can have a wider meaning. If the level of this enzyme rises it indicates increased glycolysis, a feature of cancer cells. It can also indicate the possibility of decreased aerobic mitochondrial function, another feature of cancer cells. Furthermore, at increased levels it can facilitate many of the reactions that induce increased activity and survival of cancer cells.

Pyruvate Kinase (PK) is another enzyme in the E-M pathway. This normal form of the enzyme has four protein sub-units. The altered or abnormal form, tumour marker two-pyruvate kinase (TM2-PK) has only two protein sub-units. On its own, conversion of pyruvate kinase to the TM2-PK form can have a number of causes, not exclusively cancer. However, the presence of this abnormal form of the enzyme offers corroborative evidence of the possibility of cancer when judged in conjunction with the other tests indicated and the clinical history. It is included as an optional test.

Lactic acid is produced from pyruvic acid, the terminal product of the cytosol's glycolysis pathway, when the latter is not taken up by the mitochondria. Thus, excessive production of lactic acid suggests a possible inhibition of the conversion of three-carbon pyruvic acid into two-carbon acetyl groups and the entry of these into the mitochondrial citric acid cycle. Again, this is indicative of inadequate mitochondrial function and the possibility of biochemical changes that could be leading to cancer.

Telomerase is an enzyme that acts on the telomeres or terminal sections of the DNA chains of each chromosome. This enzyme is up-regulated during times of increased and uncontrolled cellular replication as occurs in cancer.

While it is true that almost no test is one hundred per cent accurate, giving no false positives or false negatives, the results obtained by testing for one or, better, several of these compounds can be a very important component of an overall diagnostic programme and can, arguably, give a much earlier warning of an active Cancer Process than almost any other testing procedure. Furthermore, such tests are relatively inexpensive, readily available, non-invasive, other than the drawing of the blood, and non-toxic. Used as an early screening tool this First Test Panel can detect many cases of cancer long before they would be detected by other means.

As soon as biochemical errors are detected, early whole-body therapies, nutrient programmes, and lifestyle and metabolic corrections can be instigated with a good chance of the restoration of homeostasis and good health before cancer can develop further.

If these tests are abnormal, and further corroboration or diagnostic information is required, the Second Test Panel should be used. Like those in the First Test Panel, these tests are done on blood samples. They are also non-invasive and not harmful. They apply to the whole body and are not limited or restricted to single or specific tissues, organs or types of cancer. The results of this panel provide indications as to biochemical errors that can again be corrected by diet, lifestyle and the appropriate use of a wider range of natural remedies, with the similar aim of restoring homeostasis and preventing the continuation of the cancer.

SECOND TEST PANEL

The proposed Second Test Panel includes tests for important protective proteins such as p53, p21 and p185, Bcl-2, BAX, VEGF, MMP-2 and survivin and the genes that code for them.

Protein 53 (p53) is arguably one of the body's best defences against cancer, and any abnormal level of this protein, or the presence of the mutated form of it, is indicative of probable cancer. It is suggested that three tests be done: for the p53 gene in its wild or normal form, the mutated form and the protein itself.

Protein 21 (p21) is active in conjunction with p53. Both the gene and the protein can be tested for. It is suggested that they be an optional component of the Second Test Panel.

Protein 185 (p185) is produced by the p185 gene which is commonly over-expressed in breast cancer, the most common type of cancer in the UK since 1997.[53] Ninety nine per cent of it is found among women, 1% among men.

Bcl-2–associated X protein (BAX) stimulates apoptosis, vital to prevent the continuance and reproduction of faulty cells. Testing for the gene provides useful information.

B-cell lymphoma-2 (Bcl-2) gene codes for the Bcl-2 protein which counteracts BAX and is an apoptotic inhibitory protein. The balance between these two proteins is important, as well as their absolute levels.

If the level of survivin or its gene expression is high the cancer cells are likely to be particularly resistant to attack and appropriate measures should be taken to reduce this activity, possibly ahead of, and paving the way for, other treatments.

Vascular Endothelial Growth Factor (VEGF) stimulates angiogenesis, both when needed, and, inappropriately, when increased angiogenesis is required to supply blood to a growing tumour. Abnormally increased angiogenesis is indicated both by increased levels of the VEGF gene and by increased levels of an additional gene, one that codes for platelet derived growth factor (PDGF).

Matrix metalloproteinases (MMPases) stimulate the breakdown of potential target tissues. This occurs both when the fertilised embryo is endeavouring to invade and embed in the uterine wall and when cancer cells are attempting to invade distant tissues and establish a metastatic focus. High levels of gene expression of the enzymes, MMPases, are indicative of metastatic potential. There are several of these MMPases. Arguably, the level of MMP-2 is the most useful

The results of these tests, if abnormal, can indicate or confirm the probability of cancer. They will also provide indications as to the most desirable and effective correction protocols.

None of these tests are aimed at determining a location for the cancer or for a tumour. The location is important only when the therapies to be applied are targeted, physically, chemically or by radiation, at destroying the tumour. These tests detect fundamental systemic cellular changes indicative of the Cancer Process in general. They are appropriate tests when the treatment focus for recovery is on the recovery of the whole body, from the cellular level up.

CURRENT CANCER TUMOUR MARKERS

Current 'markers' for cancer are all called tumour markers, rather than cancer markers, confirming the focus of the medical system on the tumour rather than on early changes and the start of the Cancer Process. In general they are location-based, again indicating the focus of the medical approach. As such, there is no readily accepted single test that can be done on easily sampled tissue, such as blood, urine or saliva that can reflect overall body health in relation to the possible activity of the Cancer Process.

Single tumour markers do exist but are generally specific for only one type, or a limited number of types, of cancer and for specific locations. Except where specified, the following information is provided by the American Cancer Society.[54]

Bladder cancer:

"No tumour markers in urine are recommended for bladder cancer screening." The bladder tumour antigen (BTA) and the NMP22 tests can be used in combination with cystoscopy in patients who have developed indicative symptoms. These tests can be used to follow some patients after treatment, though cystoscopy and urine cytology are still recommended as the standard tests for diagnosis and follow-up. Once the cancer has advanced, other markers, such as CEA, CA 125, CA 19-9, and TPA may be elevated.

Early-stage breast cancer:

"No tumour marker has been found to be useful for screening or diagnosing early-stage breast cancer." Early diagnosis is usually based on palpation or mammogram, by which time a significantly large tumour is already present. CA 15-3, CEA and sometimes CA 27-29 are used to monitor treatment of advanced disease. Of these, CEA is the least sensitive. These markers can be used to check for recurrence but are generally thought not to be reliable for this purpose.

Chronic myeloid leukemia (CML) can be asymptomatic for several years, even when the number of leukemia cells has been increasing over time. These cells contain the abnormal gene bcr-abl which can be found in the blood and bone marrow of patients with this disease, even when it is only present in tiny amounts. A test for this gene can confirm the diagnosis of CML in a patient who is suspected of having the disease. However, CML has to be already suspected for the test to be called for.

Colo-rectal cancer:

The markers most often elevated in advanced colo-rectal cancer are Carcino Embryonic Antigen (CEA) and CA 19-9, but neither of these is considered to be useful as a screening test for colo-rectal cancer. Once a tumour is suspected and surgery planned, an elevated CEA before surgery can be used to detect a poor prognosis and to monitor treatment outcome. If the CEA is not elevated in patients with advanced or recurrent cancer, sometimes the CA 19-9 can be used to follow the disease.

Human chorionic gonadotropin (HCG) is currently accepted as the marker of choice for trophoblastic cancers and can be used to find these cancers in women who are no longer pregnant but still have an enlarged uterus.

Alpha fetoprotein (AFP) is present in foetal blood where it is a major protein, but the level normally falls soon after birth. Raised levels of AFP can occur in people with liver cancer, but it is generally only used as a screening tool in countries where liver cancer is common. It can be appropriate to use this test for people with other liver problems to detect a possible tumour, but it can also rise temporarily if there is injury to the liver.

Lung cancer:

No tumour markers have proven useful as screening tests for lung cancer, although CEA may be raised in non-small-cell lung cancer and the neuron-specific enolase (NSE) in small-cell lung cancer. However, chest X-rays or other imaging tests are usually the detection tool of choice.

Melanoma:

No tumour marker is of value in detecting early melanoma although TA-90, S-100, and some other markers can be used to test tissue samples to determine whether or not a known tumour is a melanoma. Blood levels of TA-90 have been used to detect possible metastatic spread. The blood level of S-100 is also elevated when the disease is widespread.

Myeloma:

There are no classic tumour markers that are commonly used to screen multiple or plasma cell myeloma, but tests for immunoglobulins or free light chains can be used to aid in detection or diagnosis.

Ovarian cancer:

Elevated levels of CA 125 may indicate epithelial ovarian cancer, the most common type of ovarian cancer, but is rarely raised sufficiently early to detect the cancer in time to prolong life. Other markers such as CA 72-4, CEA, and LASA-P may also be of use. The CA 125 level is not specific to ovarian cancer and may be elevated in other cancers and other conditions.

Women with germ cell tumours, the second most common group of ovarian cancers, often have elevated levels of HCG and/or AFP, which are useful in diagnosis and follow-up.

Pancreatic cancer:

No markers have yet been found to be helpful in screening for pancreatic cancer, although CA 19-9 is the most useful marker and increases with increasing spread of the disease and is useful prognostically and in patient follow-up. Measuring CA 19-9 levels can be useful in patient follow-up. Patients whose levels drop to normal after surgery have a much better prognosis than those people whose CA 19-9 remains high after surgery. This marker can also be used to follow the effects of treatment in those with more advanced disease and to watch for a possible recurrence.

Prostate cancer:

Prostate-specific antigen (PSA) is used to detect prostate cancer, although it is not specific for cancer and its presence can be due to benign prostate enlargement, inflammation or infection. It is useful for monitoring treatment and recovery. A rare type of small-cell prostate cancer has neuroendocrine features, often does not cause abnormal blood PSA, and may lead to above normal levels of chromogranin A.

Stomach cancer:

No marker has yet been developed for stomach cancer, although CEA, CA 72-4, and/or CA 19-9 may be elevated.

Testicular cancer:

Tumour markers HCG and AFP are important in testicular cancer and are used by doctors to follow its course. About 10% of men with seminoma will have elevated HCG. Some will have elevated lactate dehydrogenase (LDH), but none will have elevated AFP. More than half of men with early-stage non-seminoma disease will have elevated HCG or AFP or both. Many will also have high levels of LDH. These markers are elevated in most men with advanced disease. HCG is almost always elevated and AFP is never elevated in choriocarcinoma, a subtype of non-seminoma. In contrast, AFP, but not HCG, is elevated in another subtype known as yolk sac tumour or endodermal sinus tumour. Many tumours are made up of a mixture of different types of non-seminoma.

SUMMARY

From the above information on cancer markers issued by the American Cancer Society, it is clear that there are many markers that can be used to detect and monitor medium- to late-stage cancers or developing tumours. However, most are partially useful and in only some types of cancer. None of them can be considered to be a universal marker. In general they are aimed at the detection of tumours and not of the early stages of the Cancer Process. A panel that included tests for all of them would be unlikely to detect the Cancer Process as early as the First Test Panel proposed here and would arguably fail to detect a number of types of cancer not discussed above. Most are more useful for monitoring treatments and for prognostic predictions than for early detection. There is, currently, no generally accepted universal indicator or panel of tests, for detecting the very early stages of the Cancer Process.

PART II

EARLY DETECTION: PROPOSED FIRST TEST PANEL

Early detection of the Cancer Process is the prime focus of this thesis. This section expands the components of the First Test Panel which gives early warning signs as much as several years before a tumour can be detected.

Human Chorionic Gonadotropin (HCG)

A possible candidate for a universal and early cancer marker is human chorionic gonadotropin (HCG). Specifically, it is suggested that testing for this compound in serum or urine, or preferably both, can constitute a test that, with a significant degree of certainty can detect the early stages of many types of cancer, in many people, even before a detectable tumour has formed. For this reason it is referred to here as a cancer-process marker, rather than a tumour marker.

Gonadotropins are a group of glycoprotein hormones (GPHs) secreted by the anterior pituitary. GPHs include follicle stimulation hormone (FSH), luteinizing hormone (LH) and thyroid stimulating hormone (TSH). Chorionic gonadotropin (HCG) is produced by the placenta.

Chemically, HCG is an oligosaccharide glycoprotein with a large number of disulphide bridges and a variable molecular weight of around 37,500. It is made up of 244 amino acids[55] plus eight carbohydrate side chains. It is a heterodimer consisting of two sub-units. Variations in the carbohydrate groups account for the observed variations in molecular weight.

The alpha sub-unit consists of 92 amino acids and has a molecular weight of approximately 14,000. This sub-unit is common to all the GPHs and thus it is the same as the alpha sub-unit of LH, FSH and TSH.

The beta sub-unit has a molecular weight of approximately 23,500. It shares a 121 amino acid sequence with the beta sub-unit of LH-beta, but has an additional 24 amino acid sequence, known as the C-terminal peptide.[56] Thus, the overall beta sub-unit is unique to HCG and consists of 145 amino acids.[57]

The alpha sub-unit includes two of the carbohydrate units and the beta sub-group six. Changes in the carbohydrate units not only lead to a variable molecular weight, but the molecular weight of HCG from trophoblastic cancer is greater than that from placental HCG[58] due to the greater mass of the carbohydrate groups.[59] In combination, the two sub-units are arranged to form a small hydrophobic core within a large outer negatively-charged sphere made up of hydrophilic amino acids.[60]

HCG IN PREGNANCY

Human chorionic gonadotropin is produced during pregnancy, its level peaking at approximately the twelfth week. It is the compound that is commonly used in the over-the-counter urine test that is used to detect a pregnancy. So it is pertinent, at this point, to consider the role of HCG in embryonic development, in pregnancy, in non-pregnant or post-menopausal women, and the relevance of this in relation to cancer, both as to its presence or absence and to the amount detected.

HCG plays a major role in the successful development of pregnancy. Later it will be shown that it plays a somewhat similar role in the development of cancer.

HCG exerts its action in pregnancy via the trans-membrane receptor site LH/HCG. This is found in the cellular membranes of ovaries, testes and the uterus plus other non-gonadal tissues. It is essential for the hormonal reproduction that occurs during pregnancy, dominantly for facilitating several of the early processes of pregnancy. HCG-beta lacks the full activity potential of intact HCG. However, it is known to be a growth-promoter, increasing the growth rate of bladder cancer cells, for instance, while mouse serum antibodies to HCG-beta have the opposite effect.[61, 62]

During early pregnancy, invasive cryptoblasts secrete HCG.[63] The action of HCG on LH/HCG receptors stimulates the maintenance of the corpus luteum during the early phase of pregnancy and the production of progesterone. This progesterone then leads to a thickening of the uterine wall and the growth of the additional blood vessels required for foetal development. The vasculature of the uterus has LH/HCG receptor sites and this suggests a role for HCG in this tissue. Other tissues also have LH/HCG receptor sites with as yet undefined roles.[64]

In brief, HCG encourages and works with the actions of the trophoblasts or placental cells in establishing the pregnancy, and, as will be discussed later, ensuring the invasion of the embryo into the uterine wall, and the generation of blood vessels that will ensure a nutrient supply for the growing foetus. The capacity to both invade local tissues and develop a blood supply is clearly important at the start of pregnancy, but these two attributes are also important requirements of cancer cells and tumour development.

HCG assists the pregnancy in another way. Although the ovum is recognized as 'self' by the mother, the addition of a foreign sperm creates a 'non-self' that could be vulnerable to attack by the maternal immune system. It is thought that due to its surface negative charge HCG may reduce the action of the immune cells and increase the maternal tolerance of the 'foreign body' that is the embryo. It is thought that it does this, in part, by increasing apoptosis of T-cells.[65] This action would clearly have a detrimental effect in cancer when optimum effective levels of T-cells at the active site are required by the host for defence. A less desirable effect of the HCG produced during pregnancy may be to trigger pregnancy nausea.[66] HCG stimulates cellular differentiation and cellular proliferation,[67] activities that also have an impact on, and encourage, cancer cells and their development.

It is a contention of this thesis that the production of HCG is not only a common feature of pregnancy, but also of many different types or locations of cancer. However, there is an important difference in the level of HCG produced during a pregnancy, in which a three to four kilogram baby is expected to develop in nine months, and during tumour formation that may take many years to grow to a few hundred grams.

HCG AND EMBRYOS

A brief summary of embryo development is relevant to this discussion of cancer. It is generally accepted that cancer cells are produced every day in a healthy body. This raises the question as to how they are destroyed or eliminated. A possible answer was first suggested over a hundred and fifty years ago when it became known as the Embryonal Rest Theory of Cancer,[68, 69] proposed by Julius Cohnheim. However, little seems to have evolved from this start.

This early work was followed by the independent research of John Beard D.Sc.,[70] an English biologist who also worked in Germany and Edinburgh. He was a distinguished scientist, was honoured by the French Academy of Sciences in 1890, nominated for the Nobel Prize for Medicine in 1906 and published more than 100 scientific papers. He was the first to described apoptosis, the first to recognise the importance of the thymus gland and the first to recognise the similarity of trophoblastic cells and cancer cells.

By 1904 he was generally thought of as one of the world's leading embryologists. His research had led him to a study of the developing embryo and the similarities between placental and cancerous tissue. He stated that trophoblastic placental cells were cancer cells and developed the theory that cancer develops from 'displaced trophoblast or activated germ (stem) cells'. When he first published this work in 1904 it raised a storm of debate and gradually increasing condemnation and ridicule. In 1911 he published his book *The Enzyme Theory of Cancer* but his ideas were too far ahead of his time and of the understanding of most of his colleagues.

In the intervening hundred years a small number of people have worked with his theory. Elsewhere, Recaier in 1829[71] and Remark in 1854[72] focused on the relation of stem cells to cancer development and this became known as the Embryonal Rest Theory of Cancer.[73, 74] More recently these ideas are being rediscovered by modern medicine and thought of as the Stem Cell Theory of Cancer.

It is now recognised that as cells become differentiated their ability to reproduce or divide declines, and that fully mature cells rarely reproduce. The earlier view that cancer develops from the reproduction of mature fully differentiated cells has given way to a recognition that it develops from residual undifferentiated adult stem cells[75] or from dedifferentiated mature cells.

It is appropriate here to consider, briefly, the development of the human embryo. By the time the fertilised ovum reaches the uterus it has multiplied to a cluster or morula, of several cells. This morula has to penetrate the strong epithelial lining of the female's uterus, essentially an impenetrable wall, and then invade the tough and even stronger basal layer underneath and finally the underlying stroma or connective tissue and its blood supply.

To achieve this, the cells of the morula divide into two groups with distinct tasks. The outer trophoblastic cells must invade the uterine wall. Once that is done these cells form the placenta that protects the embryo and ensures its required supply of nourishment. When they are eventually nourished by this activity, the inner cells of the morula start to multiply further and gradually differentiate into the individual organs and tissues of the developing embryo.

One activity of the trophoblasts is to produce HCG. In health this is essentially only produced by these trophoblastic cells of the placenta. Its presence indicates that a pregnancy is occurring and it performs the functions discussed above.

The first challenge of the trophoblastic cells is to break through the epithelium of the maternal uterus. This layer of cells is strongly welded together by a variety of different adhesion proteins. To enable them to penetrate this layer the trophoblast cells produce specific projectiles or receptors on their outer cell membranes. The epithelial cells of the uterus need to co-operate with the trophoblastic cells. The epithelial cells therefore produce projections that are attracted to and bond with those of the trophoblast in firm bonds, thus achieving a starting anchorage.

The trophoblast cells secrete a range of matrix metalloproteinase (MMP) enzymes. About 24 of these MMP enzymes are known, all of which contain a metal atom in their structure. These MMP enzymes catalyse the breakdown of the ground substance of the tissue, weaken the uterine wall and enable the trophoblast to embed more deeply. When the trophoblasts reach the underlying stroma and its connective tissue, they secrete more MMP enzymes that additionally weaken this structure.

As the MMPases break down the local proteins, various peptides are produced that stimulate the fibroblasts into activity that facilitates further penetration by the trophoblasts. In addition, the MMPases from the trophoblastic cells combine with receptor proteins on the outer membrane of the fibroblasts and these in their turn start to produce more MMPases. Thus the embryo's trophoblasts and the maternal fibroblasts work together to break down the stroma.

The embryo's next requirement is a blood supply. While the developing morula consists of relatively few cells these can derive their nourishment from their surroundings, but as it grows, new cells become internalised and it has to force branches of the maternal blood supply to grow and extend capillary channels so that they divert nutrients from the mother to, and throughout, the morula.

To achieve this angiogenesis, the trophoblastic cells secrete the vascular growth hormones, vascular endothelial growth factor (VEGF), and platelet derived growth factor (PDGF). Growth of the morula within the protective trophoblastic outer layer is very slow up to this point. The embryo has been anchoring, invading, penetrating and ensuring a supply route.

The embryo has gone through these processes to and within the uterine wall, but these same processes are also initiated and accomplished by cancer cells. Cancer cells follow a similar procedure when they grow first into the primary tumour and when they metastasise to new locations. Cancer cells behave in a way that is essentially the same as that of the trophoblastic cells of pregnancy. Dr Beard put it more strongly. He stated that cancer cells behave in *exactly* the same way as trophoblastic cells and that trophoblast cells *are* cancer cells.

Once the embryo complex is securely anchored and has its own dedicated blood supply it is able to grow at a very much accelerated rate. However, in time this growth rate has to be reduced, otherwise the embryo would outgrow the capacity of the uterus and endanger the health of the mother. Choriocarcinoma would develop. Beard, around 1900, noted, and was able to demonstrate, that this enormously fast growth of the embryo slows dramatically around Day 55 of the pregnancy, around or soon after the eighth week, and that at the same time the pancreas of the embryo becomes active. He also noted that choriocarcinoma, if it occurred, started around Day 55 and that it only occurred if the embryo's pancreas failed to function. Embryonic pancreatic function is not needed for either digestion or maintenance of normal blood glucose level. Beard thus proposed that the purpose of embryonic pancreatic enzyme production at this time is to halt the rapid invasive action of the trophoblasts.

Although most of the trophoblastic cells form the placenta, Beard noted that a small proportion, some millions of them, made their way to the foetal gonads. He came to the conclusion that cancer evolves from the presence and transformation of aberrant germ cells that have lost their way en route to the foetal gonads, during embryogenesis, and become what he called irresponsible or wayward trophoblasts. He also noted that they dispersed throughout the developing foetus and formed reserve pools in all the tissues of its body. These wayward trophoblasts are what we now call adult stem cells. These adult stem cells are undifferentiated cells capable of differentiating into specialised tissue as required. They multiply symmetrically or asymmetrically.

Beard postulated that when some of the undifferentiated, or partially differentiated, tumour cells invade other tissues (metastasise) they do so by the same mechanism as that used by the developing embryo. They produce and use MMPases, they develop VEGF and PDGF and copy the activity of the trophoblast cells within the uterine wall, and in the same way they stimulate the local tissue to co-operate with them.

Once a faulty stem cell begins to multiply out of control, the host tissue actually works co-operatively with the developing cancer cells, to enable the establishment of the tumour just as it worked co-operatively with the developing embryo.

To corroborate this concept, it used to be thought that all the cancerous cells in a tumour were capable of metastasising. Now it has been shown that only about one per cent of the cells in breast tumours are capable of doing this and that these are the highly malignant stem cells.[76]

More recently, stronger links have been made and parallels drawn between foetal and cancer development and this has led to the field of oncodevelopmental biology.[77, 78]

HCG LEVELS IN PREGNANCY

Pregnancy testing uses the presence of HCG to test for the presence of an embryo.

Concentrations are commonly reported in mIU/ml where 1 IU = approx. 7×10^{-8} grams.[79]

Published detection thresholds generally range from 20 to 100 mIU/ml, depending on the laboratory and the test used.[80]

At the start of most pregnancies the level of HCG doubles every 48 to 72 hours, although this may extend to every 96 hours in the later stages. The level starts to plateau from the ninth week. This will be referred to later. The variation in the level of HCG throughout a pregnancy is shown in the table below.[81]

Pregnant women **Weeks since last period**	**mIU/mL**
3	5–50
4	5–426
5	18–7,340
6	1,080–56,500
7-8	7,650–229,000
9-12	25,700–288,000
13-16	13,300–254,000
17-24	4,060–165,400
25-40	3,640–117,000
Non-pregnant females	<5.0
Post-menopausal females	<9.5

The levels of HCG found in men and in non-pregnant women are extremely low, below the limits of detection of a much more sensitive test than the pregnancy tests. The amounts that are currently taken to be indicative of cancer by American Metabolic Laboratories are shown below and are also significantly below the limits of detection of the pregnancy tests (5–20 mIU/mL).[82]

Source of HCG or type of test	Normal level	Grey zone	Positive for cancer
Serum HCG (IRMA)	< 1.01 mIU/mL	1.0–3.0 mIU/mL	> 3.0 mIU/mL
Serum HCG (IMM)	< 1.1 mIU/mL	1.1–3.0 mIU/mL	> 3.0 mIU/mL
HCG Urine	< 1.1 mIU/mL		

Thus the normal pregnancy test is of no use for the early detection of HCG produced by cancer cells and a much more sensitive test has had to be developed.

HCG IN POST-MENOPAUSAL WOMEN

HCG levels in health, in cancer-free men and in non-pregnant women are generally below 1.1 IU/mL. However, some slightly higher levels have been found in some older but pre-menopausal women and in some post-menopausal women. This is thought to cause some diagnostic problems. To study this, Snyder and colleagues[83] examined changes of serum HCG concentrations with age in non-pregnant women and investigated the use of serum follicle-stimulating hormone (FSH) measurements as an aid to interpreting higher than expected ('positive') HCG results.

They confirmed that serum HCG concentrations in non-pregnant women increased with age and that the results were higher and significantly different ($P < 0.0001$) when compared to younger non-pregnant women. Their figures are shown below.

Age	HCG
Non-pregnant women 18-40	2.0 to 4.6 IU/L
Non-pregnant women 41-55	2.0 to 7.7 IU/L
Non-pregnant women over 55	2.0 to 13.1 IU/L

These levels are higher than the normal and threshold levels quoted by American Metabolic Laboratories and one point should be considered. Since the likelihood of anyone developing cancer in their lifetime is now over 40 per cent and since this figure rises with age, there is the real possibility that these high figures include some women with early, but as yet undiagnosed cancer. Truly cancer-free, post-menopausal women may well have a significantly lower upper limit to their HCG level than is indicated by these figures and more in line with those quoted by American Metabolic Laboratories.

When chemotherapy has been used to treat malignant tumours it may have caused gonadal suppression and a consequent rise in serum HCG to post-menopausal levels.[84] These need not indicate a regression. This can be checked by testing for serum LSH and FSH levels to see if they too are at post-menopausal levels, again due to suppression of gonad function.

HCG AND CANCERS – GENERAL

Among medical clinicians and oncologists it is generally recognised that the β sub-unit of HCG is secreted by several types of cancers. However, these are generally considered to be limited to those associated with pregnancy. Examples include gestational trophoblastic diseases such as choriocarcinoma,[85, 86] or a hydatidiform mole in which a non-viable fertilised ovum implants in the uterus. It is recognised as being secreted by cancers related to the gonads such as seminoma, a germ cell tumour of the testis, or germ cell tumours within the ovaries. In a man, a raised level of HCG is thought to be indicative of testicular cancer, particularly if it is associated with a raised level of alpha-fetoprotein (AFP). However, most oncologists, even those interested in the CAM approach, limit their expectation of the use of HCG to these cancers.

Following on from Beard's work (above), it is possible to postulate that potentially all types of solid cancers, and possibly others, produce, or are capable of producing HCG. It is now time to look at the evidence for this. If it is found, then an ultra-sensitive serum or urine test for HCG, and preferably both, could constitute an early, whole body, test capable of detecting the start of the Cancer Process, either on its own or in conjunction with a relatively small panel of tests.

The scope of the association is widened slightly by the Stanford Cancer Institute who says that, "HCG may indicate cancer in the testis, ovary, liver, stomach, pancreas, and lung."[87] According to the ARUP, National Reference Laboratory, "Increased serum HCG concentrations have ...[in addition to gynaecologically-related tumours] ...been observed in melanoma, carcinomas of the breast, gastrointestinal tract, lung, and ovaries, and in benign conditions, including cirrhosis, duodenal ulcer, and inflammatory bowel disease." This points to the possibility that either HCG can occur in totally cancer-free tissues, or that it is detecting the early stage of the Cancer Process before a tumour can be detected.

In recent years a significant body of scientific papers attesting to the connection of HCG production to a wider range of cancer types has been published. Research by many scientists and noted and acknowledged by the FDA, has shown that, "several non-trophoblastic tumours, such as transitional cell carcinoma of the bladder and urinary tract, renal cancer, prostate cancer, cancers of the gastrointestinal system, neuroendocrine tumours, lung cancer, breast cancer, gynaecological cancers, and haematological cancers, also express HCG at various levels."[88] Another study found that 25 types of human malignant tumours contained the beta chain of HCG and that it was localised both in the cytoplasm and on the surface of the malignant cells. These authors found that, "In general, it appeared that the most anaplastic or poorly differentiated cells tended to be positive, whereas well-differentiated cells in general showed a tendency to be negative [for HCG]", and conclude that, "Human chorionic gonadotropin may be responsible for both selective maternal immuno-suppression by foetal tissue and host immuno-suppression by tumours".[89]

However, even now there is little general, clinical, appreciation that HCG is produced and secreted by a much larger number of cancer cell types and that it can be used as an early warning sign of the start of these types of cancer, anywhere in the body.

The following indicates a chronological development of this concept in general and gives an indication of the variety of cancer types that have been found to secrete HCG.

In 1973 Braunstein and his colleagues reported on the ectopic production of HCG by non-trophoblastic neoplasms, and tested for it by a sensitive radioimmunoassay that measured HCG in the presence of human luteinizing hormone. These authors found that 60 of 828 patients with non-testicular neoplasms had detectable HCG. They found a high frequency of positive responses in patients with carcinomas of the stomach, liver, pancreas, and breast, with multiple myeloma and melanoma. They conclude that, "The frequency and types of tumours associated with HCG production are greater than has been previously appreciated."[90]

In 1977 HCG-positive tumours were reported to indicate a poor prognosis compared to HCG-negative tumours.[91]

In 1977, Dr Robert Williams worked with samples from the Framington study. This study started in 1948 with over 5,200 participants. It was designed as a cardiovascular study and many tests were performed on the individuals at regular intervals. Within this project serum samples were routinely taken from the participants and frozen for further study at some future date. Dr Williams studied the samples from nine patients who subsequently developed pancreatic cancer and eight who developed gastric carcinoma during the study and tested them for the presence of carcino embryonic antigen (CEA), human chorionic gonadotropin (HCG), and alpha-fetoprotein (AFP) in the time leading up to their diagnosis. He found CEA to have been raised for up to ten months prior to clinical diagnosis of cancer and HCG for up to 26 months. A single sample had raised alpha-fetoprotein but only for 10 days prior to diagnosis.[92]

Williams stated that, "Samples from 31 controls matched with the cancer subjects by age, sex, vital capacity, and smoking status showed over 20% 'false' positive CEA elevations (all smokers with low vital capacities) and over 20% borderline false positive HCG elevations in post-menopausal females." On this basis he was inclined to downplay the prognostic value of the tests. However, there are alternative explanations for the two groups. The first, the smokers etc. with raised HCG, could have started to develop cancer but as yet had no clinical symptoms of it. That, after all, is a possibility implied by the long lead time of the Cancer Process. The situation of the second group, the post-menopausal women with marginally raised levels of HCG was discussed above.

Research in 1980 on the use of multiple antigens, HCG, CEA, AFP on 253 patients with gynecologic malignancies, and on 17 patients with benign gynecologic diseases, highlighted the benefit of using at least two antigens. Plasma levels of all three antigens were significantly raised in more patients with invasive gynecologic cancers than in the control population. In this study CEA was the most commonly elevated marker, followed by AFP and HCG. Over 85% of patients with ovarian or cervical cancer had elevated plasma levels of one or more antigens prior to treatment. CEA was most often elevated in patients with mucinous adenocarcinomas of the ovary and endocervix. AFP was most often increased in patients with germ cell or stromal tumours of the ovary and in patients with large-cell non-keratinising cervical cancers. HCG was highest in patients with serous cystadeno-carcinomas of the ovary and in patients with keratinising squamous cell carcinomas of the cervix. These authors found that plasma antigen levels were directly related to tumour differentiation and stage of disease. They also found that the levels generally returned to normal eight to 12 weeks following successful therapy,[93] whereas evidence from the tests run by American Metabolic Laboratories suggests that HCG returns to normal six weeks after successful treatment.

Other authors,[94] found some cases of increased HCG after treatment, or a lack of fall in HCG. However, many treatments for gynecological malignancies involve ovarectomies. These can lead to increased production of HCG from the pituitary as it tries to trigger activity of the now non-existent ovaries. This may explain the continued increased levels of HCG.[95] This fact should be considered when assessing a patient's results.

By 1994 it was shown that cancer cells express HCG in all its forms and that HCG was consistently found in at least 85 different cancer cell lines.[96, 97]

In 1995 Acevedo et al could state that, "...cancer is a problem of development and differentiation and ...synthesis and expression of HCG, its sub-units, and its fragments, is a common biochemical denominator of cancer..."[98]

By 2004 it was recognised that expression of HCGβ by the tumours lead to increased HCG immunoreactivity in serum from patients with non-trophoblastic cancer, and that elevated serum levels occur in 30-70% of patients with most types of non-trophoblastic cancer. Furthermore, raised HCG is mostly associated with adverse outcome.[99]

By 2006 it had become clear that trophoblastic tumours containing as few as 100,000 cells could produce detectable serum levels of HCG, making it by far the most sensitive tumour marker known.[100]

Acevedo and co-workers have come up with some other interesting findings in this field. They studied cells isolated from cancer tissues and live cultured human cancer cells using analytical flow cytometry and monoclonal antibodies directed to epitopes located on five isolated sites on the human HCG molecule.[101] They found that membrane-associated HCG and its sub-units were detected from cells derived from all cancer types, irrespective of origin and conclude that it would seem that, "...the expression of these sialoglycoproteins is a common phenotypic characteristic of cancer."[102] Benign neoplasms do not express these compounds, while cultured human embryonic and foetal cells do.

To explore these findings further, they randomly selected five foetal and 28 cancer cell lines and tested them for translatable levels of HCG-beta. Single and multiple HCG6 gene activation by both the foetal cells and the different types of cancer were found, indicating that at any given time, there is the possibility of activation of as many as four of the six HCG-beta related genes.[103]

From this they concluded that cancer is a problem of development and differentiation, and that synthesis and expression of HCG, its sub-units, and its fragments, is a common biochemical indicator of cancer, and that HCG can be used not only to detect the presence of cancer cells but to determine the likelihood of metastasis. Acevedo and

Hartsock found that, "…there is a direct *in vivo* correlation between human cancer cells that metastasise spontaneously in nude mice and the expression of membrane-associated complete HCGβ (HCGβ-CTP)" and that, "Growth and local invasion *in vivo* correlates with the expression of HCG-holo."[104]

Ilkes stated that the ectopic expression of the beta-HCG is thought to occur in 20-40% of all common mucosal epithelial carcinomas where it acts as an autocrine growth factor and inhibits apoptosis. This effect may be due to its ability to inhibit the transforming growth factor receptor complex which in turn would lead to the increased risk of metastasis and to poor prognosis.[105]

Comment

There are two very important points to keep in mind when assessing these published studies on the degree of association between serum or urine HCG and the detection of cancer, and it is worth repeating and emphasising them here, particularly in view of the criticisms that are often levied at the use of HCG as a marker.

Firstly, false negatives: Many of the published papers, such as those above, use 5 IU/L or even higher as the upper range of 'normal' whereas recent research indicates that a finding of from 1-3 IU/L should be considered cause for concern and above 3 IU/L should be considered a positive indicator of cancer (See above). In addition, some of the earlier research used alternative, less sensitive, methods for determining the presence or absence of HCG, such as the Sternberger-Taylor's peroxidase-antiperoxidase technique. Thus the association between raised HCG and cancer is arguably significantly greater than the generally reported figures, using either less sensitive methods of detection and determination or a higher cut off. This is likely to be particularly true of papers reporting research done a decade or more ago.

Secondly, seemingly false positives: Since, as is postulated here, HCG could be considered to be one of the, if not the, earliest markers for cancer it is likely to detect the start of the Cancer Process before there are any other supportive signs. The assessment of this situation can only be made over time as possible progression is monitored, and I call for more research in this area.

HCG AND SPECIFIC CANCERS

Figures for the most common types of cancer, as quoted by the American Cancer Society,[106] are shown below. They have all been found to be associated with raised HCG. Tests for which could arguably have made an earlier diagnosis possible with an associated possibility of improved outcome.

Cancer Type	Estimated New Cases	Estimated Deaths
Bladder	73,510	14,880
Breast (Female – Male)	226,870 – 2,190	39,510 – 410
Colon and Rectal (Combined)	143,460	51,690
Endometrial	47,130	8,010
Kidney (Renal Cell) Cancer	59,588	12,484
Leukaemia (All Types)	47,150	23,540
Lung (Including Bronchus)	226,160	160,340
Melanoma	76,250	9,180
Non-Hodgkin's Lymphoma	70,130	18,940
Pancreatic	43,920	37,390
Prostate	241,740	28,170

Thyroid	56,460	1,780

A few examples of cancer types and related raised HCG levels are given below.

Bile Duct Cancer

Kenny and McAleer[107] report a patient with an elevated level of serum beta HCG due to cholangiocarcinoma and point out that this demonstrates the need for consideration of alternative diagnoses, other than germ-cell tumours, for a patient who presents with a raised β-HCG level.

Bone Cancer

Toshikazu Uchida et al[108] report a case of a small primary occult gastric adenocarcinoma occurring in a 57-year-old man revealing widespread metastasis to generalised bone, and associated with high serum levels of HCG and CEA as well as raised alkaline phosphatase.

Brain Tumours

Brain tissues, because of the blood brain barrier, may be thought to behave differently to other body tissues. However, cultured human cancer cells from the nervous system, including those from brain cancers, neuroblastomas, medulloblastomas and retinoblastomas have all been shown to contain membrane-associated HCG, its sub-units and fragments, as have lymphomas, leukaemias as well as all sarcomas and carcinomas studied.[109]

Primary intracranial choriocarcinoma with high levels of HCG are known to be highly malignant. Sixty six such cases showed associated tumour hemorrhage and progressive extraneural and cerebrospinal fluid metastasis. The authors felt that when the HCG level was extremely high, biopsy for histological diagnosis might no longer be needed and could increase the risk of tumour hemorrhage. To prevent this they suggest by-passing a biopsy and operating to achieve gross tumour removal followed by radiotherapy and chemotherapy.[110]

Breast Cancer

When patients with breast carcinoma were screened for abnormal concentrations of N^2, N^2-dimethylguanosine, CEA, HCG and others, the most frequently abnormal result was that of N^2, N^2-dimethylguanosine, occurring in 57% of the patients with metastatic disease. CEA levels were abnormal in 30% of post-operative node positive (N+) patients and 74% of patients with metastatic disease, while HCG elevations were found in 45% and 50%, respectively.

	Post-operative N+ patients	Patients with metastatic disease
CEA	30%	74%
HCG	45%	50%
N^2, N^2-dimethylguanosine,		57%

Other markers tested were found to be of little value.[111]

The authors found that in 13 patients with metastatic disease and an initial HCG level of greater than 5.8 mIU/ml, a fall in the level of HCG was associated with a positive response to treatment, and a rise in HCG was associated with therapeutic failure. The HCG level rose from normal to greater than 6.1 mIU/ml in six additional patients that developed progressive disease. A normal HCG level was associated with a 94.5% response rate to combination chemotherapy whereas the response rate with levels greater than 5 mIU/ml was 71.4%.

In a 1996 study, β-HCG mRNA was shown to be expressed in all breast cancer cell lines and 80% of primary breast cancers, and not expressed in negative controls. The authors conclude that expression of β-HCG mRNA, "…is a sensitive and specific method of identifying breast cancer cells in breast tissues, lymph nodes and blood."[112]

Scholl et al[113] report a case of a paraneoplastic syndrome with β-HCG production in association with squamous cell carcinoma of the maxilla and suggest that this raised HCG is consistent with the aggressive nature of the tumour.

Cervical Cancer

Many studies have shown HCG to be associated with cervical cancer.[114, 115] This is discussed later in the section on gynaecological cancers.

Colo-Rectal Cancer

Of 194 patients with adenocarcinomas of the colon (109) and rectum (85), 22.0% of colon adenocarcinomas and 21.2% of rectal adenocarcinomas showed raised levels of plasma HCG.

The level of HCG increased with decreasing differentiation, and was more common in invasive tumours (27%) than in partially invasive ones (17.1%). This follows logically from the role of HCG in establishing uterine invasion during pregnancy. The authors also found that HCG-positive tumours were more likely to be associated with liver, lymph node or peritoneal metastases, with increased CEA doubling times and with a poor prognosis. The presence of HCG was demonstrated in the dewaxed 4(mu)m sections by Sternberger-Taylor's peroxidase-antiperoxidase technique. Arguably the present day serum and urine tests are significantly more sensitive than this method and had they been used a greater correlation could possibly have been detected.

Pre-operative serum concentrations of HCG-beta were found to give more useful prognostic information than CEA in a study of 251 patients with colorectal cancer.[116]

Endocrine Tumours

A study of 360 patients with neuroendocrine tumours showed that, although serum chromogranin A is the most useful general and prognostic tumour marker for this type of cancer, not only was HCG also present but that, together with alpha-fetoprotein, this combination of three markers was clinically important, and that the latter two, when raised, indicated a poor prognosis.[117]

Gall Bladder Cancer

When tests for HCG, the free beta sub-unit (β HCG), and the core β HCG fragment (c β-HCG), measured by immunofluorometric assays in serum and urine of 29 patients with pancreatic cancer, seven patients with biliary cancer, and 45 patients with benign pancreatic or biliary diseases, it was found that β HCG showed the best diagnostic accuracy, and c β-HCG was the best marker in urine. Elevated serum beta HCG levels were observed in 72% of the patients with pancreatic cancer, in 86% of the patients with biliary cancer, and in 9% of those with benign disorders (some of whom may have as yet undetected cancers). For serum cβ-HCG the figures were 45%, 57%, and 2%, and those in urine were 55%, 71%, and 11%, respectively. The authors carry a similar caution to that offered here and state that, "Provided that they are measured by sufficiently sensitive and specific assays, beta HCG in serum and cβ-HCG in urine appear to be useful markers for pancreatic and biliary cancer."[118]

Gynaecological Cancers – General

For several decades there has been general acceptance of the fact that, if pregnancy is ruled out, raised levels of serum or urine HCG are associated with or indicative of one or more of many different types of gynaecological cancers.[119, 120, 121, 122]

Several cervical cancer cell lines have been shown to produce HCGβ[123, 124] which has also been found in tumour extracts.[125] Papapetrou et al, using chromatography techniques, found elevated levels of HCGβ in the urine of patients with cervical and ovarian cancer as well as in two with colon and esophageal cancer.

Cole et al[126] were aware that the poor sensitivity of the tests then available (1988) could be a limiting factor in using this test for routine detection of malignancy but still felt that urinary gonadotropin fragments were a promising new marker for gynecological malignancies.

Some of the patients with cervical cancer had high urinary levels of HCGβcf, detected using immunoradiometric assay and HCGβc was found to be a more sensitive marker for HCG production by tumours than serum HCG.[127] Elevated levels of HCGβcf have been detected in urine of some patients with cervical intraepithelial neoplasia.[128]

It also became clear that elevated HCG levels are associated with adverse outcome of cervical[129, 130] and vulvovaginal cancers.[131] In ovarian cancer, an elevated serum level of HCGβ has been shown to be a strong prognostic factor that is independent of stage and grade.[132]

However, even in gynaecological cancers it has been shown that a combination of markers can provide more secure information than the use of HCG on its own. When the plasma levels of HCG, CEA and AFP in 253 patients with gynecologic malignancies and in 317 patients with benign gynecologic disease were analysed it was found that CEA was most often raised, followed by AFP and HCG. Prior to treatment, over 85% of patients with ovarian or cervical cancer had elevated plasma levels of one or more antigens. CEA was most often elevated in patients with mucinous adenocarcinomas of the ovary and endocervix. AFP was most often increased in patients with germ cell or stromal tumours of the ovary and in patients with large-cell nonkeratinising cervical cancers. HCG concentrations were highest in patients with serous cystadeno-carcinomas of the ovary and in patients with keratinising squamous cell carcinomas of the cervix. Importantly, it was found that plasma antigen levels were directly related to tumour differentiation and stage of disease, and generally returned to normal eight to 12 weeks following therapy.[133]

Head and Neck Cancers

Turner et al[134] report a case of β-HCG-secreting squamous cell carcinoma of the tongue base with diffuse metastasis and suggest that HCG could be a useful diagnostic and prognostic tool.

Leukaemia and Lymphomas

HCG is not associated only with solid tumours. Lymphomas and leukaemias have been shown to contain membrane-associated HCG, its sub-units and fragments.[135] HCG has been reported in mediastinal large B-cell lymphoma[136] and in anaplastic large cell lymphoma.[137]

Liver Cancer

By 1986 it was suggested that, "HCG is one of the hormones produced by primary liver carcinoma in adults and can be localised immunohistochemically in a small number of poorly differentiated carcinoma cells."[138] HCG was known to be associated with hepatoblastomas.[139, 140]

Lung Cancer

A Japanese team describes the case of a 31-year-old female smoker, with unexplained vaginal bleeding. Tests showed HCG of 5,611 mIU/ml (normal upper limit 0.7 mIU/ml) and β-HCG of 12,238 mIU/ml (normal upper limit 0.5 mIU/ml). Right-sided chest pain led to the detection of a 12 × 10 cm poorly differentiated squamous cell carcinoma with strongly positive tumour staining for HCG. One month after right lower lobectomy and systematic lymph node dissection the serum HCG level returned to normal. The β-HCG level returned to normal at two months post-operatively and the vaginal bleeding ceased.[141] This level of HCG, while normal in pregnancy, is high in relation to cancer, however pregnancy was not detected.

An Austrian team reported a somewhat similar case. A 30-year-old female patient presented with abdominal discomfort and vaginal bleeding. Tests showed elevated β-HCG levels and led to an initial diagnosis of extrauterine pregnancy with subsequent detection of bilateral ovarian cysts. A chest X-ray then revealed a β-HCG-producing lung tumour. After resection of this the paraneoplastic symptoms resolved, and the ovarian cysts disappeared.[142]

Dirnhofer et al[143] analysed the levels of HCG, and its derivatives HCG-alpha, HCG-beta, HCG-βcf, plus LH, LH-beta, FSH, FSH-beta, placental lactogen (PL) and growth hormone (GH) in 90 patients with primary lung neoplasms made up of 40 neuroendocrine tumours, 29 adenocarcinomas, 20 squamous cell carcinomas, and one adenosquamous carcinoma. They conclude that free HCG-alpha is a useful marker for neuroendocrine differentiation in primary lung tumours, but not HCG-β.

A 68-year-old Caucasian man with generalised lymphadenopathy and numerous metastases in the lungs, liver and kidneys also had a βHCG-positive metastatic large-cell lung cancer. His serum βHCG level was 11,286 mIU/ml (upper limit of normal, 0.5 mIU/ml) and the eventual diagnosis was Stage 4 non-small cell lung cancer.[144]

Using a cut-off of 5 mIU/ml, raised levels of serum βHCG were found in 3.5% of patients with benign lung diseases and in 12% of lung cancer patients. Tumours showed the presence of βHCG in 28% of resected lung specimens. βHCG positivity was found slightly more often in adenocarcinoma than in squamous cell lung carcinoma in both tissue and serum, and most commonly in Stage 4 disease. Yet again, the response to chemotherapy was most marked in patients with the lowest levels of βHCG.[145]

Melanoma

In a study of 24 melanoma cell lines and 43 melanoma biopsies, 18 of the 24 melanoma cell lines analysed expressed beta-HCG mRNA. Melanoma biopsy specimens showed beta-HCG mRNA expression in 17 of 25 samples, and in 5 of 15 non-lymphoid melanoma metastases. The authors conclude that, "Detection of beta-HCG mRNA expression may be a useful molecular marker to define a subset of malignant melanoma."[146]

Mesothelioma

Malignant mesothelioma has been found to be associated with elevated HCG concentrations[147] in serum[148] and ascitic fluid.[149]

Myeloma

Myeloma cells have been shown to express immunoreactive HCG.[150, 151]

Ovarian Cancer

The gonadotropins influence the growth of ovarian cancer. The luteinizing hormone/human chorionic gonadotropin (LH/HCG) receptor has been found in 40% of epithelial ovarian carcinomas and it is thought that this affects the chemosensitivity of ovarian cancer cells by inhibiting apoptosis, possibly by increasing the expression of IGF-1.[152]

Parathyroid Cancer

The presence of HCG can be used to distinguish between parathyroid cancer and severe primary hyperparathyroidism caused by a benign tumour.[153]

Pancreatic Cancer

HCG or its α- and β-sub-units have been proposed as specific quantitative markers for malignant pancreatic endocrine tumours.[154]

In a study of 36 patients with exocrine pancreatic adenocarcinoma, 12 patients with chronic pancreatitis, and 21 healthy controls, 40 per cent of patients with pancreatic adenocarcinoma and only one patient with chronic pancreatitis had detectable plasma concentrations of βHCG (p<0.01). Furthermore, these patients had a statistically significantly worse outcome than those with no detectable βHCG.[155]

157 pancreatic endocrine tumours from 155 patients were tested for α- or β-sub-units of HCG by immunocytochemistry. HCG-α-immunoreactive cells were found in 75% of functioning malignant pancreatic endocrine tumours and in one of 67 functioning benign tumours, in one of 17 non-functioning malignant and in none of 17 non-functioning benign tumours. No β-HCG-immunoreactivity was localised in the tumours. The authors conclude that, "HCG-α appears to be a reliable quantitative and qualitative marker for malignancy in functioning pancreatic endocrine tumours."[156]

Alfthan et al[157] found that, provided sufficiently sensitive and specific assays were used, βHCG in serum and cβHCG in urine were useful markers for pancreatic and biliary cancer.

Type of disease	Raised serum βHCG	Raised serum cβHCG	Raised urine cβHCG
29 cases of pancreatic cancer	72%	45%	55%
7 cases of biliary cancer	86%	57%	71%
45 patients with benign pancreatic or biliary diseases	9%	2%	11%

This points to the wisdom of utilising more than one form of HCG as markers; in this case, serum and urine forms of βHCG. In other studies αHCG was found to be more reliable.[158]

Louhimo et al[159] studied the prognostic value of tumour markers CEA, CA 19-9, CA 242, CA 72-4, and HCGβ in serum. HCGβ was measured by immunofluorometric assay based on monoclonal antibodies specific for the free β-sub-unit of HCG. While CEA was the most commonly raised marker they found that HCGβ, followed by CA 72-4, and the stage of the cancer were the strongest independent prognostic factors in this study. It would have been interesting to know the values for the other components of HCG and for the results from urine tests.

Kahn et al[160] did measure the sub-units of HCG, and did so in 76 patients with pancreatic islet-cell tumours. They found that 17 of 27 patients with functioning islet-cell carcinomas had elevated plasma levels of HCG or one of its sub-units (HCG-α and HCG-β), compared to none of the 43 patients with benign disease or the six patients with non-functioning malignant tumours.

Prostate Cancer

Sheaff et al[161] analysed prostate tissue from transurethral resections from 80 consecutive cases of adenocarcinoma of the prostate. Beta HCG was detected in 12 cases, nine (75%) of whom had metastasis and 11 (92%) of whom were dead in 18 months. Of the 68 βHCG negative cases, 21 had developed metastases (31%) and 25 (37%) had died within 18 months. In the βHCG negative group there was an association between histological grade and survival but none was found in the βHCG positive group. Testing for βHCG on its own can give some information but is not adequate as a stand-alone test.

Stomach Cancer

A number of early studies report the association of HCG with cancers of the stomach.

Focal HCG was found in association with scirrhous argyrophilic cell carcinoma of the stomach in three of 59 patients, in 1982.[162] A 57-year-old man with a small primary occult gastric adenocarcinoma and widespread metastasis to generalised bone had associated high serum levels of HCG, CEA, and alkaline phosphatase.[163]

Thyroid Cancer

Sagauchi et al,[164] studying the effect of ectopic HCG from a papillary thyroid cancer cell line on rat thyroid cells, found that ectopic HCG possesses intrinsic thyroid-stimulating and growth-promoting activity. They state that the ectopic HCG may act as an autocrine-paracrine factor in non-trophoblastic neoplasms. See also case history of RY at the end of this thesis.

Urinary Tract Cancers

HCG is known to be a growth-promoter, increasing the growth rate of bladder cancer cells. As would be expected from this, antibodies to HCG-beta from mouse serum have the opposite effect.[165, 166] However others, in 1996, found HCG a less useful marker.[167]

Endogenously produced beta-HCG by bladder tumours *in vivo* has been associated with a poor prognosis, suggestive of an autocrine or paracrine beta-HCG-induced stimulation of tumour growth.[168]

Jenkins et al[169] found that β-HCG in bladder cancer indicated resistance to radiotherapy, as did Moutzouris et al.[170] Oliver et al[171] showed that HCG positive bladder cancer responded less well to chemotherapy.

Dobrowolski et al[172] found that β-HCG was a good biological marker to differentiate between superficial and deep urinary bladder tumours.

A 60-year-old man with painful gynaecomastia and polycythemia was found to have a β-HCG-secreting clear renal cell carcinoma. By six months post-radical nephrectomy his gynaecomastia had regressed and his serum β-HCG level had become undetectable.[173]

A 23-year-old male was diagnosed with urothelial carcinoma, with trophoblastic differentiation of the bladder. The carcinoma contained giant cells that were positive for HCG.[174]

SUMMARY

From the foregoing it is clear that HCG is associated not only with choriocarcinoma of pregnancy, but also with all gynaecological cancers. This is generally accepted by the medical profession.

Furthermore, it is clear from research studies that HCG is associated with almost all the common cancers. Unfortunately these associations do not seem to have penetrated clinical centres. A desirable outcome would be to find that HCG levels are raised in all types of cancers and in all cases. So far this has not been shown, but more research is required.

However, many of the studies showing only low to moderate associations were done using less sensitive analytical methods than are available and in common use today. As further studies are reported, in which increasingly sensitive analytical tests are used, it is probable that HCG may be found to be associated with all types of cancer to a greater or lesser extent. The association may become even more apparent when there is greater recognition that a lower reference level than was used in many of the above studies is appropriate. As discussed elsewhere, provided that CAM therapies and not MDS ones are instigated, the danger following a false negative result is greater than the danger of a false positive.

The results discussed above also point to the benefit of using more than one marker for detecting the start or presence of the Cancer Process, and, if further corroboration is required, the use of the further tests described in this First Test Panel, and the Second Test Panel discussed later.

TESTS FOR HCG

HCG exists in a number of forms and these can be detected in body fluids such as serum and urine. It can be present as:

* free intact HCG;
* free alpha sub-units, HCGα;
* free beta sub-units, HCGβ;
* partially degraded fragments such as:
  * nicked HCG (HCGn);
  * nicked free HCGβ (HCGβn);
  * other HCG-like substances (HCGLS).

The nicked forms of both HCG and HCGβ are cleaved at different points between amino acids 44 and 48 and may be present in the serum of patients with cancer as well as the other forms.[175] There may also be some HCG without the C-terminal peptide (CTP) in the urine of some people with cancer.[176]

The analysis of body fluids for HCG goes back to 1927 when Ascheim and Zodek tested for its biological activity in urine as a test for pregnancy.[177] In time this bioassay and its modifications were replaced by immunoassays.[178, 179] With the availability of monoclonal antibodies it became possible to test for the individual sub-units of HCG and to use the results for detecting not only pregnancy and trophoblastic cancers but also non-trophoblastic cancers.[180] The most clinically relevant forms were eventually identified as intact HCG, its sub-units HCGα and HCGβ, the partially degraded or nicked forms of HCG (HCGn) and HCGβ (HCGβn), and the beta-core fragment (HCGβcf).[181] There are also some other glycosylated forms. Clearly there has been a lack of standardisation as to the nomenclature of the various fragments; however their identity has generally been clear. Stenman et al[182] have sought to improve this.

READILY AVAILABLE TESTING FOR HCG

In the 1950s, through the work of D. Manuel Navarro and Dr Howard Beard, a Yale-trained biologist and chemistry professor, the Anthrone Colour Test was used to detect HCG.[183] The test was done on a urine sample. However, this test did not discriminate between the alpha and beta sub-units but only indicated total HCG-like components.

More recently it has become possible to determine physiological levels of HCG in both urine and serum. The test uses a monoclonal antibody and is specific for the beta sub-unit. This sub-unit is unique to HCG and avoids giving a false positive by detecting the alpha sub-unit that is also present in FST, LH and TSH.

In most medical laboratories beta HCG is determined by chemiluminescence or fluorimetric immunoassay[184] with a limit of detection between 5 mIU/ml and 20 mIU/ml. This is fully adequate for pregnancy testing but is not sufficiently sensitive to detect the start of the Cancer Process.

In 1980 Dr Emil Schandl of American Metabolic Laboratories started the development of his CA Profile.[185] Initially the panel consisted of three tests, those for HCG-beta, PHI and CEA. Using that test the results showed that, "94% of patients (n=133) with proven cancers displayed at least one abnormal result... and ...26% of patients without proven cancer (n=197) displayed one or more elevated tumour markers. A number of these 'false positive' results were in individuals with signs or symptoms of cancer (e.g., enlarged lymph nodes, breast lumps, etc.), but without pathologic diagnoses. Some were later diagnosed with cancer."[186] Thus, these so-called 'false' positives were in fact indicative of very early Cancer Process and not false at all, but time driven. Any report of raised HCG should provide triggers to encourage the individual to take better care of their health and hinder or reverse the Cancer Process.

The test panel from his laboratory subsequently grew to include two forms of HCG in serum: IRMA HCG and IMM HCG. Later a third test was included, for HCG found in a urine sample and labelled HCG-U. When only the two serum test results are used there remains a small possibility of false positive results caused by non-specific heterophilicimmune binding HCG fragments or HCGLS. This grouping of three HCG tests offers a much more secure test with very much less likelihood of producing either false positives or false negatives.

- The IRMA HCG result derives from a test done by an immunoradiometric assay and detects only the intact HCG molecules, none of the fragments or separate sub-units.

- The IMM HCG result is obtained by chemiluminescence and detects not only the intact HCG molecules, but also the sub-units and fragments and the HCGLSs. Thus, the IMM result is usually higher than the IRMA result.

- The urine test, done by chromatographic immunoassay, includes all HCG forms except for HCGLS. A positive result for HCG-U reduces the risk of the final assessment being based on a false positive due to the presence of HCGLS.

HCG (IRMA and IMM) can be measured in serum. The blood is allowed to clot, then centrifuged and the clear serum drawn off. This is done before it is sent to the testing laboratory. As serum is more stable than whole blood, transport is easier and less time dependent. Samples can be sent from different countries and have been found to give reliable results for up to two weeks.

Some laboratories rely only on urine HCG but this too is open to errors if it is used as the only test for HCG.

Three tests on urine samples exemplify this. DS (a case history referred to later) had a urine test for HCG several months after surgery. Her first result of 56 IU came from a laboratory that quoted 1-49 IU as normal. Several months later her result was identical. This is a surprising consistency in itself, not seen in more recent tests quoted later. It is also surprising in that she had followed an aggressive CAM treatment programme in the interval. Further doubts were raised when a friend of hers, in good health, agreed to submit a sample for comparison and this too came back at 56 IU. This raised some doubts as to the validity of the results from that laboratory and certainly about relying on only one test. The third result is unlikely to be a true positive as the friend is still well many years later.

With increasing age of the individual there is the possibility of developing gonadal insufficiency with consequent decreased output of oestrogen or testosterone. In response there is increased pituitary output of LH and FSH, and as a result a small output of HCG-like substances that are common to LH, FSH and TSH. These do show up in the urine but clearly their presence is not related to trophoblastic or cancer cells. By assessing the levels of IRMA-HCG, IMM-HCG and HCG-U in combination it is possible to make a more secure assessment of the results and to avoid chasing after false positives.

CONSEQUENCES OF HCG ACTION

HCG not only indicates that the Cancer Process is active and there is a developing cancer but it facilitates the process. Further, it indicates its degree of aggressiveness and its invasive potential. As in pregnancy, HCG reduces the power of the immune system to damage or destroy either the embryo or the developing cancerous tumour respectively. It has been suggested that HCG changes both the cell-mediated and the humoral immune response to the stimulus of cancer antigens,[187] and that the HCG on the tumour surfaces suppresses the action of the T-cells and increases their apoptosis.[188] In this way it stimulates proliferation and local invasions.[189]

By the late 1980s it was known that raised levels of HCG in patients with malignancies was associated with a high level of invasiveness[190] and a poor prognosis.[191] Jenkins et al[192] found that beta-human chorionic gonadotropin in bladder cancer indicated resistance to radiotherapy, and Oliver et al[193] showed that HCG positive bladder cancer responded less well to chemotherapy.

In a 1989 study Iles et al[194] measured βHCG in 127 urine and 85 serum samples from 175 untreated patients with urothelial cancer. The results are in the table below.

	Localised (restricted) disease	**Patients with widespread metastasis**
Serum βHCG significantly raised	2 of 64 patients (3%) Disease confined to the pelvis.	16 of 21 patients (76%)
Urine βHCG moderately raised	11 of 25 patients (44%) Locally advanced disease.	5 of 7 patients (71%)

They conclude that, "Measurement of serum and/or urine βSHCG appears to be an efficient diagnostic marker for the presence of distant metastases in bladder carcinoma." (βSHCG indicating β-serum HCG.)

HCG was measured in 100 patients with transitional cell carcinomas of the bladder who were treated by transurethral resection of the tumour. All patients received a course of radical radiotherapy, with salvage cystectomy for those who failed to respond; 51% did not respond to treatment. Pre-treatment tests included staining for HCG which, in combination with the amount of observed squamous differentiation, proved to provide the best prognostic outcome of treatment. Other histological features studied included the grade of tumour necrosis, inflammation, vascular invasion, and growth pattern but these were found to be unrelated to each other or to clinical outcome.[195]

Their results are shown below:

Tumours	Failed to respond to therapy
With areas of squamous differentiation	47 of 60 (78%)
Staining positively for HCG	22 of 29 (76%)
Both features	22 of 23 (96%)

Other authors[196] have also found that not only is HCG a useful indicator of the presence of cancer cells, it is an indicator and harbinger of worse to come. HCG and HCGLS inhibit immune activity, increase motility and angiogenesis,[197] inhibit apoptosis in general,[198] and stimulate metabolic, regulatory, growth and cell proliferation in target cells and organs, thus increasing the possible development of any type of cancer. These may seem to be inappropriate actions for the host, but it should be kept in mind that this activity is designed primarily to support and help the developing embryo. If it is happening in tumour formation this is, arguably, a fault of the host in not controlling the tumour development.

HCG is an autocrine proliferative factor as it will cause the replication of the cell within which it is made, such as trophoblasts, stem cells and cancer cells.

Many other studies have shown that a raised HCG level is consistent with a worsened prognosis, for instance in pancreatic cancer[199] the level of HCG indicates how metastatically aggressive a tumour may be. "Neither non-embryonic cells nor benign tumour cells express HCG, but HCG-beta is a defining phenotype statement of malignant transformation."[200]

One author[201] has concluded that treatment of breast cancer in rats with raised HCG-beta may induce apoptosis, and in another study inhibition of HCG-beta has been shown to induce apoptosis in choriocarcinoma cells.[202] The latter authors conclude that, "...HCG, through its binding to the LH/HCG receptor, may augment proliferation and inhibit apoptosis in choriocarcinoma JAr cells..."

Butler and Iles[203] endorse the contentions made here, that the ectopic production of free HCGβ is a common phenomenon in epithelial tumours and they add that HCGβ may significantly affect tumour development by inhibiting apoptosis and thus increasing cell populations. They suggest that HCGβ may produce this effect by "...antagonistic inhibition of other cystine knot growth factor receptors." They go on to point out that, "...there are structural similarities and it has been thought that HCGβ could interfere with the growth-inhibiting effect of transforming growth factor β (TGF-β), platelet derived growth factor (PDGF) and nerve growth factor..."

The level of HCG can rise within days of cancer cells developing, within days of the individual moving from Phase One (pre-cancerous) to Phase Two (the presence of cancer cells) of the Cancer Process. This can occur a long time, possibly many years, before a tumour is of sufficient size to be detected. There is considerable evidence that an abnormal level of HCG, even if it is only small, generally leads on to a tumour in the future, possibly months or sometimes years ahead.

Measuring HCG post-surgery can indicate whether or not 'they got it all, and you do not need further treatment'. According to Dr Schandl at American Metabolic Laboratories, "After successful surgery, provided all of the tumour has been removed and there are no metastatic foci, the markers should be negative in three to six weeks, depending on the extent of the surgery."

Thus, establishing the levels of HCG pre- and six weeks post-operatively can help to indicate the degree of success of the surgery. Future tests can also be used to monitor the possibility of a recurrence. Pre-operative levels can also indicate the probability of metastasis and of aggressiveness. Further, monitoring HCG levels can indicate the probable success of any treatment programme.

It is unfortunate that the general clinical response, at the moment, to any suggestion of testing for HCG is that, "HCG is only present in choriocarcinoma, the type of cancer which can occur during pregnancy, and is of no relevance in any other type of cancer." This seems to be the generally held MDS wisdom, and much preventive work is hindered by this assumption.

Using 85 different cancer cell lines, intact HCG has been found in cell membranes in association with metastatic aggressive tumours of many different histological types and origins, and in the blood and urine of patients with bladder, gastrointestinal tract, lung, and skin (melanoma) cancers and others as well as in embryonal carcinomas,[204, 205] and cancer of the lung, pancreas and liver[206, 207, 208] and rarely in benign cells. Even when detected in healthy people it may be an indication of a very early stage of the Cancer Process, as yet undetected by less sensitive means. It therefore seems likely that raised levels of HCG or PHI (see below) may be associated with all types of cancer, in line with the trophoblastic origin of cancer postulated by Beard. Certainly, any indication of a raised level of HCG should be taken very seriously and responded to accordingly.

HCG is an autocrine proliferative factor that will cause the replication of the cell in which it is made, such as trophoblasts and stem cells, and cause them to proliferate. Similarly, PHI, which will be discussed next, is now recognised as autocrine motility factor.

Mitochondrial Function

THE WARBURG EFFECT

Nobel Prize winner Dr Otto Warburg, back in the 1930s, believed that the ultimate cause of cancer resided in the mitochondria. He stated that it was a failure or uncoupling of the electron transport chain and compromised oxidative phosphorylation at the cellular level.[209] Healthy cells have an absolute requirement for oxygen. Cancer cells can live without oxygen and can thrive in a low-oxygen, anaerobic or anoxic environment. This is a critical distinction between the two cell types. Cancer cells can derive a major proportion of their energy from substrate phosphorylation, either or mostly from the cytosol's Embden-Meyerhof (E-M) pathway, or alternatively from substrate level phosphorylation or amino acid fermentation in the mitochondria. Healthy cells derive almost all of their energy, as ATP, from the aerobic citric acid cycle and then via oxidative phosphorylation and the electron transport chain, both of which occur within the oxygen-rich mitochondria.

Warburg postulated that the lack of oxygen caused healthy cells to revert to an increased dependency on glycolysis and the E-M pathway for energy production and thus become cancer cells,[210] stating that, "...the cause of cancer is no longer a mystery, we know it occurs whenever any cell is denied 60% of its oxygen requirements"[211], and "Cancer, above all other diseases, has countless secondary causes. But, even for cancer, there is only one prime cause. ...the prime cause of cancer is the replacement of the respiration of oxygen in normal body cells by a fermentation of sugar."[212]

Every time Dr Warburg put healthy cells in a controlled laboratory environment and totally deprived them of oxygen he found that they had turned into cancer cells. They reverted back to being undifferentiated cells, eminently capable of repeated uncontrolled replications and multiplying to form a tumour. With an adequate supply of oxygen they reverted back to aerobically functioning healthy cells. Modern research continues to prove Warburg's theory.[213]

An alternative theory is that it is fundamentally mitochondrial damage, rather than oxygen deprivation, that leads to cancer.[214] Tumour mitochondria are also structurally damaged. However, it is known that if mitochondria are deprived of oxygen for any extended period of time they suffer irreversible damage.[215]

Gatenby and Gillies point out that increased glycolysis, even in aerobic conditions, is a common feature of both primary and metastatic cancer cells, leading to increased cellular dependency on, and uptake of, glucose. They propose that this is an adaptation to intermittent hypoxia in pre-malignant lesions. This increased glycolysis leads to local acidosis and so to evolution of phenotypes that are resistant to acid-induced cell toxicity. These cells then have a strong growth advantage which leads to proliferation and invasion.[216]

Seyfried[217] carried these ideas forward and gives evidence for mitochondrial failure and impaired electron transport chain and the resulting disordered energy metabolism as the ultimate cause of cancer. He states that aerobic glycolysis, arising from damaged respiration, is the single most common phenotype found in cancer, and that (a) the absence of oxygen leads to anaerobic glycolysis which leads to the production of lactic acid; and (b) tumour cells with damaged respiration experience aerobic glycolysis which also leads to increased output of lactic acid, but this increased level of lactate is persistent in cancer cells.

Cells that can adapt to intermittent failure of the electron transport chain by increasing their level of glycolysis (and hence of PHI, see below) can survive and become cancer cells. Cells that fail to adapt in this way die.

The electron transport chain, oxidative phosphorylation and an appropriate supply of oxygen come together in healthy mitochondria. When this link breaks, the result is the formation of cancerous cells. There is also evidence that a high level of oxygen has the opposite effect and inhibits the growth of cancer cells.[218]

Thus, electron transport chain failure is a fundamental cause of cancer. It can be caused by any number of epigenetic factors (labelled 'carcinogens' as a result) that adversely affect mitochondrial function. It can also be induced or aggravated by mutated genetic factors that, it is now proposed, are themselves the consequences of cancer rather than its cause.

Early signs of the Cancer Process can therefore include evidence of increased glycolysis in the cytosol and a sustained increased level of lactate.

Embden-Meyerhof Pathway (Glycolysis)

Pasteur, in 1857, noted that when a yeast-rich liquid was exposed to increased oxygen the fermentation rate decreased but cellular growth increased. Yeast can produce energy either by anaerobic glycolysis leading to pyruvate with the production of 2 ATP molecules, or, when the oxygen supply is increased, by conversion of pyruvate to acetyl CoASH which is then metabolised via the aerobic citric acid cycle with a production of 32 ATP molecules. This became known as the Pasteur Effect.

Dietary complex carbohydrates are broken down to glucose in the digestive tract. This enters the bloodstream, then enters cells where it is metabolised in the cytosol to pyruvate via the E-M pathway. Other sugars, such as fructose or galactose, are transported to the liver and converted to glucose, which then follows the same pathway. Each molecule of glucose releases 36 molecules of the high energy compound ATP. Thirty two of these are released in the oxygen-rich mitochondria via the citric acid cycle followed by oxidative phosphorylation via the electron transport chain. The other four are released via substrate level phosphorylation via two possible pathways. One of these is the E-M pathway. The other is via the succinyl-CoA synthetase step of the mitochondrial citric acid cycle. This pathway is more important under anaerobic than aerobic conditions when oxidative phosphorlyation dominates.

The cytosol-based E-M pathway of glycolysis consists of nine steps. Glucose is first converted to glucose-6-phosphate, a step that requires energy and phosphate (as ATP). It is catalysed by glucokinase. Glucose-6-phosphate is then rearranged to fructose-6-phosphate in a reaction catalysed by phosphohexose isomerase (PHI), to be discussed shortly. This is followed by a second step that requires energy and phosphate (ATP), this time catalysed by phosphofructo kinase. This last step is irreversible and rate-limiting. The remaining steps involve cleavage of the six-carbon sugar into two three-carbon molecules, dihydroxyacetone phosphate and glyceraldehyde. These are eventually converted to two molecules of pyruvate.

Most of the energy of glycolysis is harvested, in the cytosol, by the conversion of nicotinamide adenine dinucleotide (NAD) to the reduced and higher-energy form, NADH. Each molecule of NADH has the potential of generating three molecules of ATP, but, and in the case of cancer this is problematical, only if there is on-going oxidative phosphorylation activity in fully functioning mitochondria where the three molecules of ATP can be harvested and the NADH converted back into NAD within the electron transport chain.

The alternative method of regenerating NAD occurs in the cytosol and involves the conversion of pyruvate to lactate, a reaction catalysed by lactate dehydrogenase. This reaction leaves the NAD available in the cytosol to harvest more energy and convert to NADH, but, although lactate is a high energy molecule, it does not provide a significant amount of useful, readily available cellular energy. In fact, the lactate has to be transported out of the cell and processed by the liver. See later.

Thus, cancer cells are energy challenged. They depend on large amounts of readily available glucose from which they can only derive a very small amount of the available energy, and they produce large amounts of lactic acid.

PHOSPHOHEXOSE ISOMERASE (PHI)

PHI (phosphohexose isomerase) was discovered in 1933 when it was noted that, "...a significant correlation was found to exist between the phosphohexose isomerase and alkaline phosphatase activities in the sera of patients with cancerous disease."[219] It has since been shown by many authors to be raised in people with a variety of types of cancer. It is an enzyme worth exploring and requires more research.

PHI is one of a family of multifunctional phosphoglucose isomerase proteins and it plays several distinct roles. Within cells, in the cytosol, it is involved as a catalyst in glycolysis and gluconeogenesis. Specifically it catalyses the reversible isomerization of glucose-6-phosphate and fructose-6-phosphate as indicated above.

In the extra-cellular environment it is a neurotrophic factor for spinal and sensory neurons. It may also be a molecular messenger. It is produced and secreted by leukocytes, and acts to regulate the growth of several different cell types.

It is secreted by cancer cells, from which it acts as an autocrine motility factor,[220] stimulating metastasis,[221] stimulating angiogenesis and inhibiting apoptosis.

AUTOCRINE MOTILITY FACTOR (AMF)

A cell motility-stimulating factor was isolated from human, serum-free A2058 melanoma cells in 1986[222] and labelled 'autocrine motility factor' (AMF). It was described as being a protein of 55kDa with a high content of serine, glycine, glutamic acid, and aspartic acid residues. It was shown to stimulate the motility, either random or directed, of the producer cells but not to attract neutrophils and not to be replaced or blocked by known growth factors such as epidermal growth factor. Large amounts were shown to be produced in three different clones of ras oncogene-transfected metastatic NIH 3T3 cells but not by the non-transformed parental cells. Thus it was suggested that it might play a major role in the local invasive behaviour of individual tumour cells and might facilitate the concerted invasion by groups of tumour cells into healthy tissues.

The structure of AMF was determined in 1990.[223] It was shown to be the previously cloned cytokine and enzyme known either as neuroleukin or phosphohexose isomerase (PHI) and this was confirmed when specific PHI inhibitors, such as carbohydrate phosphates, inhibited the enzymes' activity and AMF-induced cell motility. These authors note that PHI had already been implicated in cell motility, and found to be a marker of cancer progression.[224]

PHI/AMF acts via the tumour autocrine motility factor receptor site, gp78. This is a transmembrane protein, an ubiquitin protein ligase, located on the endoplasmic reticulum. Its expression is positively correlated with tumour metastasis.[225]

It is increasingly becoming clear that AMF and PHI are identical; however both names continue to be used, interchangeably and confusingly, in the literature. It is also clear that increases in the level of serum PHI/AMF are positively correlated with increased cancer risk and with increased risk of metastasis. "Autocrine motility factor (AMF), which is identical to phosphohexose isomerase (PHI)/glucose-6-phosphate isomerase (GPI), a ubiquitous enzyme essential for glycolysis, neuroleukin (NLK), a neurotrophic growth factor, and maturation factor (MF) mediating the differentiation of human myeloid cells, enhances the motility and metastatic ability of tumour cells."[226] These authors found that both raised serum PHI/AMF and increased gp78-expression were needed for the increase in motility and metastatic ability.

The level of PHI/AMF secretion and the expression of its receptor (also known as AMF R) are closely related to tumour malignancy. AMF signalling has been shown to induce anti-apoptotic activity. Human fibrosarcomas that secrete high levels of AMF have been shown to be resistant to drug-induced apoptosis[227] and thus are non-responsive to many forms of chemotherapy.

In addition, highly AMF-expressing HT1080 cells have been shown to induce aggressive angiogenesis *in vivo*. The expression of a vascular endothelial growth factor (VEGF) receptor was enhanced in AMF-expressing tumours dependent on protein kinase C and phosphatidyl inositol 3 kinase (PI3K) activation.[228]

In 2007, Funasaka and Raz[229] reviewed the role of AMF and tumour environment on malignant processes. Confirming it as a tumour-secreted cytokine, abundant at tumour sites, they describe it as a "...multifunctional protein capable of affecting cell migration, invasion, proliferation, and survival..." and comment that it has phosphoglucose isomerase activity.

Baumann et al[230] measured the serum PHI level in 435 patients with malignant gastrointestinal, kidney, and mammary tumours prior to primary treatment and in 181 patients with benign diseases and disorders and reported the results shown below:

Cancer type	Sensitivity	Specificity
Gastrointestinal and kidney	70%	92%
Early stages without metastasis	60%	
Mammary	40%	

They therefore suggest that determining serum PHI can be a useful tool in monitoring gastrointestinal and renal cancers.

It is clear that many transformed or trophoblastic cells with increased glycolysis produce and secrete increased amounts of PHI and that the blood level of this enzyme correlates with the aggressiveness of many forms of cancer.

Comments

The level of PHI can be elevated close to the start of the Cancer Process or when an active tumour is present. However, it is important to note that it can also be elevated in some other conditions. It can be raised immediately following a heart attack or severe muscular trauma or in severe hypothyroidism (not low-grade chronic hypothyroidism), in AIDS[231] or viral hepatitis.[232] In relation to the latter it has been compared to other enzymes including: aldolase, isocitric dehydrogenase and pyruvic transaminase[233] and used in the differential diagnosis of liver disease.[234]

If none of the above conditions apply and if serum PHI is above normal levels it could be indicative of an active Cancer Process: in head and neck cancers,[235, 236] cervical cancer,[237] breast cancer,[238] and gastrointestinal cancer[239] and many others. The presence of raised serum PHI was found to be a more useful indicator than two other enzymes, alkaline phosphatase or glutamic oxaloacetic transaminase, in detecting early lung cancer.[240] It has been found to be useful in screening healthy women for cervical cancer during a mass cytology programme.[241] Baumann and colleagues found it to be "a useful indicator in the preventive check-up of gastrointestinal and renal cancer."[242] In head and neck cancers serum PHI levels increased with the advancing stage of the disease and gradually decreased following radiotherapy.[243]

The level of PHI in the blood can rise for as long as fourteen years before there is a conventional tumour diagnosis[244] and thus detecting an early increase provides a useful early warning marker.

CONSQUENCES OF RAISED PHI

A raised level of serum PHI is indicative of increased E-M pathway or glycolysis activity in the cell's cytosol, and so of the possibility that the cell is turning or has turned anaerobic and cancerous. But that is not all. Raised PHI has implications for the increased progression of the Cancer Process. Raised levels have further negative consequences. When AMF was found to be the same as PHI[245] the authors stated that: "AMF was detected in a major proportion of lung carcinomas, and may play a part not only in proliferation and/or progression of the tumours, but also, possibly, in the differentiation of squamous cell carcinomas."

AMF (PHI) inhibits apoptosis.[246] When AMF-affected cells were inoculated into mice, tumours formed, the cellular replication rate doubled and there was increased resistance to apoptotic agents.[247] There have been other reports of AMF- (PHI-) induced resistance to apoptosis. When, for instance, the anti-cancer apoptotic drug mitomycin C was used, the AMF-affected cells were found to be resistant to it.[248]

Many compounds lead to, or stimulate angiogenesis. This process is needed not only for wound healing and tissue replacement and repair, but for the growth of the additional blood vessels that are needed by a tumour to feed the individual cells within it. Angiogenic factors include fibroblast growth factor (FGF), tumour necrosis factor (TNF)-alpha, transforming growth factor (TGF)-beta and vascular endothelial growth factor (VEGF).[249, 250, 251] The most important of these is VEGF,[252, 253] and AMF has been found to increase the production and activity of VEGF,[254] thus increasing the potential for the development of tumour-directed blood vessels.

Raised levels of PHI (AMF) can cause yet a further problem. Either directly or indirectly PHI increases tissue permeability and increases the risk of abdominal ascites.[255] Thus, an increased level of serum PHI both suggests that cells have turned cancerous, and that the further development of cancer is being encouraged by decreased apoptosis, increased angiogenesis and increased risk of metastasis.

Dr Schandl of American Metabolic Laboratories has suggested that the biochemical initiator of metastasis is PHI (AMF), and that elevated plasma levels of PHI may lead to metastatic events such as cytokinetic vibration and dislodgement of the cancerous cell from its neighbouring environment with consequent embolism via lymph or blood flow to distant sites.[256]

TUMOUR MARKER 2-PYRUVATE KINASE (TM2-PK)

The enzyme pyruvate kinase (PK) catalyses the last step in the E-M pathway, the conversion of phosphoenol pyruvate to pyruvic acid, which in turn is the precursor to the acetyl groups within the mitochondria. Magnesium is essential for the function of this enzyme, but its activity is hindered by calcium. This last step in glycolysis is one of the three rate-controlling steps of the pathway.

The inactive form of pyruvate kinase is converted to the active form when the ratio of blood insulin to glucagon is high, which in turn happens when the blood glucose level is high. Conversely a low ratio of these two hormones inhibits the production of the active form of pyruvate kinase.

The normal form of pyruvate kinase has four protein sub-units. An altered and abnormal form of this enzyme is known as tumour marker 2-pyruvate kinase or TM2-PK. It is similar to pyruvate kinase (PK) but has only two protein sub-units instead of the normal four. It is produced in increased amounts by undifferentiated cells or proliferating tissues, including a number of cancer cell types. Its production is thought to be due to the different metabolic requirements of cancer cells. Specifically, it enables cancer cells to use a metabolic shortcut that saves energy which is then used for cellular replication.[257]

An increase in the amount of TM2-PK in the blood can indicate a variation in the activity of the normal E-M pathway. Raised levels of TM2-PK have been found in the blood of people with solid tumours and this test has, for instance, been used with considerable success to distinguish between benign and malignant cervical tumours.[258] TM2-PK has also been found in lymphocytes, and in lymphoproliferative disorders.[259] The level of TM2-PK has been shown to increase with disease progression and tumour stage in lung cancer,[260, 261] and it has been suggested as a better marker than CA19-9 and CEA in gastrointestinal cancer.[262]

Comments

However, like PHI, TM2-PK is not raised solely in cancer cells.[263] The amount present can also be increased in other conditions where there are problems of abnormal cellular glucose metabolism. So although this test is helpful, it is even more useful if the results are viewed in conjunction with the results of all the other tests. It may be a less useful component to the proposed panel of tests than PHI, which appears to play a greater role in the encouragement of the Cancer Process.

ACETYL CoASH

All the reactions of glycolysis, to this point, have occurred in the anaerobic cytosol. At this step in the breakdown of glucose there are two options. Firstly, and desirably, pyruvate is converted to acetyl groups in a reaction catalysed by pyruvate dehydrogenase, an enzyme dependent on the coenzymes vitamins B1, B2, B3 and lipoic acid. The acetyl group is then combined with CoASH, a vitamin B5-dependent enzyme, in a fully irreversible reaction that occurs on the inner surface of the mitochondrial membrane. I have referred to this in *Cancer Concerns* as a pivotal step as it is critical to healthy, aerobic cellular metabolism and the avoidance of cancer. There are several reasons for this.

Firstly, anaerobic cancer cells derive their energy almost entirely from glucose. This glucose is not produced, *de novo*, from within the cells but must be obtained from the diet. It is important that proposed beneficial changes to lifestyle and diet do nothing to increase the level of glucose available to cancer cells.

Secondly, most fats and amino acids are metabolised to acetyl groups and to acetyl CoASH, which then enters the mitochondrial citric acid cycle. Because the conversion of pyruvate to acetyl CoASH is irreversible, the CoASH produced by the catabolism of fats or proteins is not converted to glucose within the body. Thus, a low carbohydrate diet with a high content of above ground, high fibre, low carbohydrate vegetables, plus good quality oils and fats and some proteins, otherwise known as a ketogenic diet, is an excellent way to reduce the amount of glucose available to tumour cells. It has been suggested that the level of intake of protein be only moderate, as some of the amino acids can be converted to glutamine which may be a useful energy source for tumour cells.[264]

Within the healthy mitochondria, the acetyl groups, as acetyl CoASH, derived from fats, proteins or carbohydrates, are degraded round the citric acid cycle, releasing energy, carbon dioxide and water. The energy, in the form of NADPH, NADH and FADH, is broken down, energetically and converted, via oxidative phosphorylation and the electron transport chain, to ATP.

A few cells, such as red blood cells, do not have mitochondria and rely almost totally on glycolysis for energy. Cancer cells, which commonly have faulty electron transport chains in their mitochondria, obtain almost no energy from the fats, which release their energy via the activity of healthy and oxygen-rich mitochondria, and very little from dietary proteins, although some can be obtained via substrate-level phosphorylation from glutamine in the mitochondria.

If that all-important initial step is obstructed, and the pyruvic acid cannot be converted to acetyl groups and then to CoASH, it is converted instead, in an energy dependent step, to lactic acid. This pivotal reaction can be hindered by a lack of several nutrients, including vitamins B1, B2, B3, B5, biotin, lipoic acid and magnesium. It will also be blocked if there is mitochondrial damage or loss, as occurs in cancer cells.

LACTIC ACID

Pyruvic acid is the end product of glycolysis, the cytosolic anaerobic breakdown of glucose via the E-M pathway. It can be converted into a number of compounds. Under normal aerobic conditions it is converted into acetyl CoASH which enters the citric acid cycle. It can be converted back to glucose, by gluconeogenesis via a different reverse pathway, and it can be converted into the amino acid, alanine. Under anaerobic conditions it is converted to lactic acid in a reaction catalysed by lactic dehydrogenase.

Healthy and very active muscle cells can produce amounts of pyruvate faster than can be processed by their mitochondria and the available oxygen. This leads to a build-up of lactic acid. This is not processed within the cytosol of the muscle cells and but leaves the cell by facilitated diffusion attached to a specific transport protein in the sarcolemma. This is a slow process and when lactic acid is produced rapidly it will accumulate in the cell, reducing the pH. Osmotic forces then dictate a flow of water into the cell which leads to swelling congestion and, in turn, possible reduced capillary circulation due to this congestion.

Lactic acid is a high energy molecule, containing 619 Kcal, almost as much as glucose which has 686 Kcal. This can be released, elsewhere in two ways. One of these is by oxidation. The heart, for instance is highly aerobic. During exercise, when the overworked muscles are producing lactate, the heart has a high energy requirement and a ready supply of available oxygen, and so can utilise the lactate. It is oxidised back to pyruvate and re-processed, via the heart's mitochondria.[265]

Secondly, lactate can be metabolised via the lactic acid cycle and gluconeogenesis, mostly in the liver. This is a slow process by which two lactate ions are rebuilt back into glucose, using energy in the form of ATP. In fact, more energy is used in rebuilding the glucose than was extracted during glucose conversion to lactate, thus there is a net energy loss with each circuit of this cycle.

However, cancer cells have developed a use for lactate and thrive on it as an additional energy source. At the start of tumour formation the cells can acquire their oxygen from existing blood vessels. As a tumour increases in size it triggers the production, via vascular endothelial growth factors and related mechanisms, of new capillaries. Inevitably, some cancer cells are closer to a supply of oxygen than others. Overall there is a reduced supply of oxygen to tumours than to healthy tissues.[266, 267] Whereas it had been thought that normoxic tumour cells primarily use glucose for oxidative energy production, it is now known that lactate is a substrate that fuels the oxidative metabolism in such cells.[268] Hypoxic tumour cells primarily use glucose for glycolytic energy production and release lactic acid waste product, creating an inverse relationship between lactate and oxygen levels.

Cancer cells do produce large amounts of lactic acid. It had been assumed that, as a result of poor vascularity, this was due to an inadequate supply of oxygen. It was then suggested that the cause was dysfunctional mitochondria,[269] which takes us back to the ideas of Warburg.

Lactate accumulation in human tumours is associated with increased risk of metastasis, increased risk of tumour recurrence, and poor survival.[270, 271, 272] By increasing the mast cells output of angiogenic factors it is also a risk factor for increased angiogenesis.[273]

As summarised in a review by Hirschhaeuser, Sattler and Mueller-Klieser:[274]

* Increased glucose uptake and accumulation of lactate, even under normoxic conditions, is a common feature of cancer cells.
* Lactate-induced secretion of hyaluronic acid by tumour-associated fibroblasts stimulates metastasis.
* Lactate induces the migration of cells and cell clusters.
* Radioresistance has been positively correlated with lactate concentrations.
* Lactate facilitates immune avoidance by cancer cells.
* Lactate bridges the gap between high lactate levels in wound healing, chronic inflammation, and cancer development.
* Lactate induces secretion of VEGF.

From this it is clear that a persistent and tumour-derived increase in blood lactate level is indicative of an active Cancer Process and that it leads to increased immune avoidance, angiogenesis, metastatic potential, reduced (MDS) treatment success, and a poor overall prognosis.

Raised levels of lactic acid can, therefore, be considered a risk factor. For this reason serum lactate levels are included in this First Test Panel to detect early signs of cancer and indicate a therapeutic goal.

Carcino Embryonic Antigen (CEA)

Carcino embryonic antigen (CEA) has been discussed earlier, along with various tumour markers and in relation to HCG, AFP and other factors. It merits a brief discussion here.

CEA is a glycoprotein. More specifically it is a glycosyl phosphatidyl inositol (GPI)-cell-surface anchored glycoprotein that is produced and active during the development of the foetus where it is involved in cell adhesion.

Cell adhesion molecules are proteins embedded in and through the cell membranes. They are involved in bonding both between the cell and the surrounding extracellular matrix, and between its own cell and a neighbouring cell. CEA plays an important role in foetal growth and development, but its production usually stops before birth takes place.

It is thought that tumours that spread via the bloodstream produce or use CEA to help them adhere to healthy cells such that they can anchor to a new location, and thus it encourages metastasis.[275, 276, 277]

CEA, in any significant amount, is not normally present in the blood of healthy people, with the exception of heavy smokers, in whom it may presage a future cancer. Although generally thought of as a marker for colon cancer, it has been found in the serum of people with cancer of the breast, colon, lungs, pancreas, rectum, stomach and thyroid medulla. Further research may show it to be associated with other types of cancer. Somewhat like HCG, levels of CEA, if raised, should return to normal within about six weeks of surgery or other successful treatment.

CEA can be raised in conditions other than cancer, including Crohn's disease, cirrhosis of the liver, pancreatitis, and ulcerative colitis. However, here, as with smokers, it is possible that this could be an early indicator of a future cancer potential.

When 35,000 plasma samples from more than 10,000 patients and healthy subjects from approximately 100 institutions were analysed for CEA and the results assessed it was considered by Hansen et al that the assay was, "...of value as an adjunct in the diagnosis and management of the cancer patient", and that, "A progressive increase in the CEA level ...was of unfavourable prognostic significance."[278]

However, Ando et al[279] tested seven possible cancer markers, including CEA, AFP, CA19-9 and CA 125, on 300 patients with non-small-cell lung cancer, of which 200 patients had adenocarcinoma and 112 squamous cell carcinoma. They found CEA to be the most useful for adenocarcinomas, showing 45% positivity for adenocarcinoma patients, a result that improved with severity of disease. However, this does indicate its limited value, on its own, as an indicator of the start of the Cancer Process before there are other symptoms.

Some years ago I read a medical report on the possible use of the measurement of CEA to detect a recurrence of cancer after the removal of a tumour of the colon and part of the colon itself. The paper's author then made the comment that there seemed to be little point in running this blood test as it would not provide information as to the location of the tumour, and that it would be better to wait until a new tumour had grown to sufficient size that it could be detected, and then it could be worked on. This is typical tumour-focused thinking. From the CAM perspective this test offers the obvious benefit that it warns that the Cancer Process is operative and that greater effort has to be put into correcting the metabolism. Essential lifestyle changes can then be made, aimed at preventing any further deterioration.

Because a raised CEA level can indicate other errors and not just cancer it is important, yet again, that these results be considered in association with the results of the other tests suggested in this thesis, to enable a more accurate overall assessment to be made. If the level of CEA has been high when a primary tumour was first detected and then falls post-treatment, it has been shown that a future increase in CEA level could be indicative of a possible reoccurrence of the Cancer Process and the need for greater therapeutic activity.[280, 281]

Comment

In brief, CEA is normally absent in the blood. It can be raised in a number of health problems but particularly cancer, and if it is indicative of cancer it is most commonly indicative of cancer of the colon, but can be due to cancers elsewhere. Thus, on its own it is of limited value, either prognostically or as a progress marker. However, it has its place in a panel of tests such as is proposed here. In combination with HCG, PHI and lactic acid it provides an increased chance of avoiding false negatives.

Telomerase

Cancer cells reproduce very much faster than healthy cells. One method of detecting or confirming the beginning of Phase Two of the Cancer Process, the promotion and progression of cancer cells, is based on measuring any increase in the rate at which cells reproduce.

Telomeres are lengths of non-coding DNA, made up of repeating nucleotides (TTAGGG) that occur at each end of each chromosome, prevent adhesion of the chromosomes, and protect the ends of the DNA chains. During chromosome replication there is a necessary loss of part of the terminal chain, specifically of one or more of the telomeres, with each replication. After a specific number of copies of the DNA helix have been made, usually several thousand, the Hayflick limit is reached, when there are no more telomere segments left. The chromosome ends are no longer protected and thus become damaged, and the cell can no longer produce healthy daughter cells. This is a natural aging process at the cellular level and requires the action of protein 53 (p53), a tumour suppressor protein (see below). Without this control, cells would keep dividing, endlessly, a feature of cancer.

Telomerase can be active in the nucleus, where there is nuclear DNA (nDNA) and also in the mitochondria where there is mitochondrial DNA (mDNA). It can also be detected in the blood as extra-cellular telomerase.

In cancer, ongoing cancerous cell proliferation is achieved by bypassing the Hayflick limit. This is achieved by suppressing the activity of protective p53 and another protein, retinoblastoma protein or pRb. Some of these cells are then, with the help of increased activity of the enzyme telomerase, able to rebuild their telomeres and continuously replace the ones that are lost. The cells thus become immortal and able to replicate endlessly and build ever-growing tumour masses.

To achieve this outcome extracellular telomerase enters the cell's nucleus and switches on the c-myc oncogene which in turn stimulates the expression of the cell's own telomerase and acts on the cell's DNA. C-myc is a proto-oncogene. Under normal conditions it regulates the growth and proliferation of cells. When it is mutated, present in excessive amounts, or is over-activated, it becomes an oncogene and stimulates excessive telomerase activity and thus increased potential for cell growth and proliferation. It is frequently present, mutated or in abnormal amounts, in people with cancer.

It has been suggested that telomerase located in the mitochondrion plays a protective role by decreasing mitochondrial levels of reactive oxygen species (ROS), whereas nuclear-located telomerase stimulates excessive telomere building.[282] This could then mean that mitochondrial dysfunction is associated with decreased levels of protective mitochondrial telomerase and stimulates cancer development as a result.[283] Put another way, a relative increase in nuclear telomerase stimulates cellular replication; a relative decrease in mitochondrial telomerase allows for increased damage due to ROS.

Telomerase does more than protect telomeres. It stimulates glycolysis, thus increasing the energy available to cancer cells.[284] When its activity was blocked the activity of 73 genes was reduced,[285] including some that stimulate tumour growth. Further, there was evidence that inhibiting excessive telomerase activity in cancer cells also reduces their metastatic potential.

Several factors or mutations, in combination, can lead to the conversion of a healthy cell into a tumour cell via the activation of its telomerase. These include:

1. Over-activation of TERT (telomerase reverse transcriptase).
2. Reduced production of p53 (see below).
3. Loss of pRb, a tumour suppressor protein that, in health, blocks inappropriate activity of the cell cycle. It can be inactivated by proteins such as are produced by the human papillomavirus (HPV). When this happens, the cell cycle and cellular reproduction can continue unabated, contributing to tumour growth, particularly, but not only, in the cervix.
4. Activation of Ras genes. These genes carry signals from the extracellular environment into the cell and to the cell's nucleus where they code for cell growth, differentiation and survival. Mutations of the Ras family of genes are the most common form of mutation or proto-oncogenes.[286] If they do become mutated they can be left permanently switched on and thus they become oncogenes and can contribute to cancer. In general they are found in twenty to twenty-five per cent of cancers but can be found at much higher levels in certain types of tumours.[287]

Telomerase is rarely active in mature healthy cells and any such activity is generally low and not sufficient to lead to excessive telomere replacement and longevity. It is active in some types of white blood cells in which longevity and replication are important.

There are two possible sources of telomerase. Intra-cellular telomerase is produced by the cell itself and found associated with nDNA and mDNA. It is needed, in health, by certain cells where on-going reproduction is important. These include some of the cells of the immune system, hair follicle cells, germ cells and stem cells.

Extra-cellular telomerase comes from outside the cell. It enters the cell, migrates through the cell's cytosol and enters the nucleus where it can both act on its own and can stimulate the cell's own telomerase activity. It has been suggested that extra-cellular telomerase can derive from a retrovirus.[288] Extra-cellular telomerase can also be derived from other cancer cells that have been destroyed.

Telomerase activation has been detected in up to 90 per cent of tumours,[289] which suggests that it plays a vital role in the rapid growth and development of cancer. The remaining cells, those that do not utilise telomerase to ensure their immortality, are thought to have found an alternative method, known as the alternative lengthening of telomerase (ALT) mechanism.[290]

Approximately three quarters of women with breast cancer, including ductal carcinoma *in situ*, have raised telomerase levels, and it has been suggested as an early marker of the development of breast cancer. [291]

The level can start to rise as cancer starts to develop and can be above normal even before a detectable tumour is formed. This means that a positive test for an abnormally raised level of intra-cellular telomerase can be an early warning sign for cancer. The level can also be used to monitor a treatment plan. If successful, the intra-cellular telomerase should fall back to normal.

A high level of extra-cellular telomerase can have several meanings. It may indicate an active Cancer Process. It may also be due to telomerase having been released from dying cancer cells, possibly following successful treatment, or from viruses.

It is worth noting that the level of telomerase activity has been shown to have increased following psychological stress. Patients showed an increase of 18 per cent in telomerase activity in peripheral mononuclear cells after an hour of acute stress.[292] It is widely recognised that cancer often follows a period of great or prolonged stress.

However, it has also been suggested that telomerase plays a positive role by protecting mitochondria when under mild stress.[293]

CYP1B1

CYP1B1 is one of the large group of cytochrome P450 enzymes. It catalyses many reactions including those relating to the metabolism of cholesterol and other steroids, and those relating to the metabolism of a number of drugs and several procarcinogens.[294]

It has recently been suggested as an early systemic marker for cancer. It is said to be unique to cancer cells and its presence indicative of any type of cancer anywhere in the body.[295] It has been further suggested that it stimulates the conversion of inactive plant ingredients, salvestrols, into compounds that are specifically toxic to the cancer cells that produce it. It has been argued that since non-cancerous cells do not contain CYP1B1, the salvestrols (phytonutrients) in foods and supplements are not converted into cytotoxic agents in healthy cells and thus these healthy cells are not harmed by the salvestrols. The salvestrols are almost ubiquitous in a vegetable and fruit rich diet and thus available for defence against cancer when a vegetable and fruit rich diet is consumed.

If CYP1B1 becomes accepted as a fundamental test for the early detection of the presence of cancer it will be important to discover how early this detection is possible and how that compares with the early detection achieved by the First Test Panel suggested here. This will clearly take many years to establish. The long-term early warning aspect of the First Test Panel has already been established, based on approximately thirty years of testing.

There is a fundamental difference between the two approaches. An HCG-PHI-CEA-lactic acid panel looks for early changes in cellular biochemistry and metabolism that could lead on to cancer but may not yet be due to fully-developed cancer. This is particularly true of increases in PHI and lactic acid. These changes start before, and probably contribute to, the development of fully cancerous cells. Thus, by its very nature, this panel of tests provides an important early marker of possible adverse metabolic changes as well as of changes that are already established. This may not be something that can be achieved by testing for CYP1B1.

Summary of Proposed First Test Panel

There is general agreement and good evidence that, as with any health problem, the sooner any aberration from normal is detected and efforts are made to correct this, the more likely it is that a successful outcome be achieved. Arguably, up to 93 per cent of all cancers are diet and lifestyle related.[296] Even for people who argue with this high estimate, few would argue with the contention that well over half of all cases are so related. We know that dietary errors such as the intake of sugar, refined carbohydrates, trans fatty acids, over heated fats, hydrogenated fats and oils, nutrient deficient foods, food additives in all their many forms, and an acid residue diet increases the risk of cancer. We know or suspect that many of the common lifestyle habits increase our intake of toxins and carcinogens. Yet few people choose to make positive changes, seeming to assume that 'cancer will not happen to them'.

The cure rate for cancer is appallingly low and the treatment unpleasant or worse. Most people endeavour to ignore it until such a diagnosis is forced upon them. A simple test, or panel of tests, that has a high chance of detecting cancer soon after the first cells have turned cancerous and long before a detectable tumour has formed, offers many advantages. Such a test would enable people who are so minded to make positive and healthy changes to their diet and lifestyle and 'back-off' from the full development of cancer, thus avoiding the possibility of being subjected to the trauma of medically imposed surgery, chemotherapy and/or radiation that generally follows from a biopsy-confirmed diagnosis of cancer.

It is suggested here that the panel of tests, consisting of HCG, PHI, telomerase, lactic acid and CEA, could provide such an early warning. These tests, albeit by different laboratories, are currently available and each has had a significant history of research and development. Their use should be actively encouraged and promoted. The finding of any values that lie outside the normal range should encourage the individual to make serious but non-invasive early changes in their lifestyle. Such actions could save their lives.

It is worth noting the results of a reduced panel of tests, including only HCG (in three forms), PHI and CEA, as reported on the website of America Metabolic Laboratories:[297]

"Dr Schandl's *Cancer Profile©* produced more persuasive percentages; this panel has an impressive accuracy of 87-97%. Looking at three cancer markers together (HCG, PHI, CEA), 221 positives in 240 breast cancer patients (92 per cent) were detected. Of lung cancer patients, 127 of 129 (97 per cent) were correctly diagnosed. And with colon cancer patients, 55 positives out of 59 patients (93 per cent) were correctly identified."

False Negatives and False Positives

Very few medical tests are perfect. The functioning of the human body is too complex for that. There are almost always some false negative results, where detection is missed, or false positive results where a problem is thought to exist when in fact it does not. Before planning a testing protocol it is important to understand these facts in relation to the tests being performed, the use that will be made of the results, and the possible consequences of any such errors.

In this regard it is important to emphasise that a large component cause of cancer is made up of the individual's errors of diet and lifestyle. The level of causation ranges from ultra-conservative figures of around 60 per cent to as high as 95 per cent.[298, 299] It has also been said, by Craig Venter, one of the first to sequence the human genome that, "Human biology is actually far more complicated than we imagine. Everybody talks about the genes that they received from their mother and father, for this trait or the other. But in reality, those **genes have very little impact on life outcomes**. Our biology is way too complicated for that and deals with hundreds of thousands of independent factors. **Genes are absolutely not our fate**. They can give us useful information about the increased risk of a disease, but in most cases they will not determine the actual cause of the disease, or the actual incidence of somebody getting it. Most biology will come from the complex interaction of all the proteins and cells working with environmental factors, not driven directly by the genetic code."[300]

This being the case, cancer can be regarded as a lifestyle-induced preventable disease and not genetically dictated, as has been misguidedly promulgated. This leaves the individual largely in control. They can do much to improve their diet and minimise the harmful aspects of their environment and lifestyle. However, many people need some evidence that changes in their current diet and lifestyle are needed; otherwise there is the inclination to follow the 'it can't happen to me' syndrome. Thus, a potential test for the earliest possible indication of cancer is useful. If it is positive, even if, by definition, no other symptoms are present and a tumour not yet located, diet and lifestyle improvements are going to be, or should be, the first step in any recovery or correction protocol. These are non-harmful protocols with no unwanted toxic effects. They also offer many positive other health benefits in addition to the avoidance of cancer and other inflammatory conditions.

In a medical system that applies treatments such as surgery, chemotherapy and radiation, all of which have high levels of risk and adverse or toxic effects, including the triggering of cancer itself, it is important to avoid tests that can give false positive results, such as mammograms.

In a healthcare system that aims at restoring normal function with treatments that are beneficial to the body and in harmony with its normal and healthy function, not only are toxic effects avoided, but false positives are less of a problem. At worst they may trigger some anxiety, but equally they can be triggers for the individual to improve their diet and lifestyle, and arguably could improve their general health even if the person does not have cancer. Such has commonly been the case in this author's practice. In this situation it is more important to focus on the avoidance of false negative results and the failure to detect early signs of the problem and so to fail to take preventive measures.

Bearing in mind that such tests may well be the earliest sign of cancer a seemingly false positive, a positive result unconfirmed by other tests, could merely be due to the fact that the indicated test result is indeed the first sign of possible cancerous changes and not at all 'false'.

FALSE POSITIVES

Testing biological systems presents its own problems. As yet there is no simple single test for the presence of cancer that is one hundred per cent reliable.

The reasons for this include daily physiological changes, genetic variations, epigenetic factors and parameters unique to each individual that can affect the composition of any sample tested. There is the accuracy of the sample collection and identification, of the test itself and of the interpretation based on the result. The many different types of cancer cells can behave differently.

With a test panel such as is offered here, it is helpful to look at the subject from a broader perspective.

The Cancer Process is one of progressive degeneration, first at the biochemical and cellular and then at the physiological and tissue levels. Whereas in many other health problems, reversal and cure are possible, and normal health can often be restored by reversing the causes, the situation in relation to cancer is more complicated.

For instance, it is hypothesised[301] that, whatever the final trigger, cancer is made more likely following a period of stress, particularly of the 'helpless and hopeless' variety. This leads to adrenal exhaustion, reduced microcirculation, reduced oxygen to the tissues, reduced mitochondrial function, glycogen engorgement at the cellular level, increased anaerobic cytosol metabolism, increased levels of PHI and the production of l-lactic acid which can then increase the risk of mitosis.[302] This process cannot be reversed simply by removing or leaving the stressful situation. Much more has to be done to restore adrenal health, mitochondrial function and a return to normal cellular function.

For these and many related reasons it is very much easier to reverse the Cancer Process close to the start rather than after it has become more firmly established, and so early detection is vitally important. Detection of raised levels of the components of the proposed First Test Panel offers a tool by which this can be achieved.

In Relation to HCG

If pregnancy is excluded and the cautious allowance made for small rises in HCG levels in post-menopausal women, HCG is a very sensitive tumour marker in most types of cancer. However, any such result should always be considered in relation to the overall result of multiple tests before a conclusive diagnosis of cancer is made. If a raised level of serum HCG is the only problematic result, urine levels should always be checked. This avoids the possibility of detection of forms of HCG, which are not excreted in urine,[303] as previously explained. Even so, some false positives are possible and have, in the past, in medical practice, led to needless and harmful surgery or chemotherapy.[304, 305] If the serum level of HCG is low the urine result may show negative if the urine is very dilute. A repeat test should resolve this.

A number of physiological factors can lead to a false positive result. While it is assumed that HCG is only produced by placental or malignant cells, there is some evidence of the production of small amounts by non-malignant tissues. An HCGβ-like substance with little or no carbohydrate was detected using a radioimmunoassay and a radioreceptor gonadotropin assay in extracts of liver and colon obtained at autopsy from three patients who died of non-neoplastic disease. The authors suggest that, "...the genome responsible for the [HCG] production is not completely suppressed in adult nonendocrine tissues."[306]

Braunstein[307] suggests that these false positive results include the presence of pituitary HCG, or luteinizing hormone and non-human chorionic gonadotropin. A false positive could be due to interference by anti-animal immunoglobulin antibodies. These latter include heterophilic antibodies and species-specific antibodies derived from dairy and other animal products, or other contact with animals, such as human anti-mouse antibodies which can be used in the test procedure. Other factors include complement, non-specific serum factors and anti-HCG antibodies.

False positives can also occur within the laboratory. These include exchange of samples, carry over by pipetting and other techniques, and labelling errors. Errors can result from the presence of fibrin clots in serum as a result of incompletely clotted specimens, interference from other endogenous components in the blood such as bilirubin, haemoglobin, and lipids,[308] or the presence of heterophile antibodies, human anti-animal antibodies, rheumatoid factor, and autoantibodies.[309]

If a positive result is due to cancer the level of HCG will generally rise over time, thus a second test a few weeks after the first can help to clarify the significance of the data.

It is worth noting that most HCGβ is catabolysed to HCGβcf during excretion into urine.[310] Thus, if a raised serum HCG level is due to HCGβ, its concentration in urine will be low. It may not be detected if the serum HCG result is only slightly raised, as most tests for HCG do not measure HCGβcf.[311]

Similarly, as detailed elsewhere, a raised level of PHI, while indicating a probable increase in anaerobic activity within the cytosol, may have causes other than cancer, and the same is true of CEA and lactic acid.

However, when the proposed tests are combined into one panel, as suggested here, and several of the results are indicative of the start of the Cancer Process, such a diagnosis becomes more secure. Yet, as always, there is, at least theoretically, the possibility of both false positives and false negatives.

Comment

To summarise and expand this discussion, there are several possible causes of false (non-cancer) positive results for raised HCG. They include:

* elevated levels of pituitary HCG;
* perimenopause;
* chemotherapy-induced suppression of gonadal function;
* previous injection of HCG;
* interfering substances such as:
    * anti-animal Ig antibodies, heterophilic antibodies, and species-specific antibodies;
    * rheumatoid factors;
    * complement;
    * non-specific serum factors;
    * anti-HCG antibodies.
* assay problems:
    * sample exchange;
    * carry over from pipettes and other devices;
    * labelling problems.

The dangers of acting on the base of a possible false positive result are immense if this is taken as an absolute assumption of cancer and the application of allopathic conventional medical strategies, dominantly surgery, chemotherapy or radiation, is instigated as these three strategies pose considerable risks and high levels of long-term toxicity and damage to health.

It is this author's view that no toxic treatment should be started solely on the basis of the conventional tests for blood markers or, even, of the tests discussed here. In the case of this panel of tests this is particularly true given that such a positive result would still not indicate a possible location of any suspected cancer and the majority of medical treatments are tumour location focused.

A paper entitled *False-Positive HCG Assay Results Leading to Unnecessary Surgery and Chemotherapy and Needless Occurrences of Diabetes and Coma*[312, 313] might seem to be denigrating the HCG test. As such it is worth considering here. Six women tested positive for HCG (up to 451 IU/L). They were referred to gynaecologists, but ultrasound, laparoscopy, dilation and curettage showed no evidence of recent or current pregnancy. Four of the six 'positive' cases had been detected and followed with the Abbott Diagnostics AxSym HCGβ test and one of six had been followed with the Abbott Diagnostics IMx HCGβ test, designed for detecting pregnancies.[314] The tests detect intact HCG, non-nicked or bioactive HCG, HCG free β-sub-unit and HCGβcf at three concentrations. Two positive serum results were obtained but HCG, free β-sub-unit, or HCGβcf (<3IU/L) were detected in parallel urine samples. Trophoblastic disease or post-gestational choriocarcinoma was suspected, though the results were later labelled 'phantom' and thought to be attributable to human anti-mouse IgG or to heterophilic antibodies. Five of the women were given chemotherapy, two underwent a hysterectomy and another an oophorectomy. One developed Type-I diabetes and became comatose. If invasive or toxic therapies are to be applied, a biopsy-proven cancer is clearly a more secure diagnosis although the biopsy itself poses risks, including that of increased risk of metastasis. Had these women been given a panel of tests, such as suggested here, it would probably have been found that all the other components were negative, since they are not related to the subsequently presumed causes. Had they then been prescribed supportive CAM therapies instead, these false positives might have caused anxiety, as must have occurred in this example, but, as the HCG levels finally subsided these concerns would also have subsided, and their general health may well have improved.

Two more comments are pertinent. Firstly, as will be obvious from earlier figures, these levels are far above those found in cancer, where 3 IU/L (5.8 IU/L in some studies) is taken to be positive for cancer. Secondly, urinary HCG forms are included in the proposed test panel to reduce the possibility of false positives.

It is worth emphasising again that the situation, in relation to false positives in general, is somewhat different when CAM therapies are on offer. These therapies are not aimed at tumour destruction by toxic or risky means. They are aimed at working sympathetically with the body and restoring it to normal function by means of improving the diet and lifestyle, detoxing, supplying all the nutrients needed by the body, and particularly the mitochondria, correcting problems such as adrenal exhaustion, blood glucose level imbalances, hypothyroidism, diminished immune function, the presence of *Candida albicans* and other moulds and pathogens, and more. All of these strategies will improve general health, even if the HCG level is a false positive. The corrective strategies can all be followed as part of a prevention strategy by anyone wanting to avoid cancer and, if the test results are high and truly indicative of the start (or progress) of the Cancer Process, rather than a false positive, these strategies can help to start reversing the process.

Thus, while it is always desirable to aim for the best possible accuracy and validity of any test and its results, the dangers resulting from a false positive result are far less when a CAM procedure is being followed. Since this test is for very early warning signs, corroborative evidence may not be available and such results may indeed turn out, in time, to be true positives. Any positive test result should be monitored over time, as such symptoms and evidence could well develop if corrective strategies have not been put in place.

It can be argued, particularly if CAM strategies are being used for early correction, that it is more important to avoid a false negative result from a test or panel of tests, and miss an early diagnosis, than to avoid a false positive.

Biopsies versus these Tests

A biopsy, with clear evidence of cancerous cells, is generally considered to be the final indicator of the presence of cancer, or malignant tumour. However, there are disadvantages and dangers associated with doing biopsies. The comparison below indicates some of the benefits of the test panel suggested here, over a biopsy.

Biopsy Advantages	Biopsy Disadvantages	Advantages of the HCG-related First Test Panel
The type of malignancy can determined.	Biopsies are impractical as a general screening tool and not possible until there is a tumour.	The test can be used as a screening tool as all that is needed are blood and urine samples.

The location of at least part of the tumour, the part that was extracted for biopsy, can be determined.	Biopsies are location-specific; they are not a general guide, or early warning, as to whether or not there are cancerous cells anywhere else in the body.	The test is a general guide as to whether or not there are cancer cells anywhere in the body.
	Taking the tissue sample can be painful or inconvenient.	Drawing blood is simple and relatively painless. Collecting urine is completely painless.
If the biopsy has involved total removal of the tumour this may contribute to a 'cure'.	Waiting until there is a significant tumour to sample is leaving things too late for early intervention.	The existence of only a few cancer cells can be detected within six to ten weeks of their formation.
Testing a biopsied sample can indicate the degree of the malignancy at that location.	Biopsies give no information about other locations, even relatively close by.	The test provides information in relation to your whole body.
	When tissue is taken for biopsy, cancer cells can be released from the local site and metastasise to another tissue.	Drawing blood does not increase the risk of metastasis.
	A biopsy cannot be used after surgery, to establish whether or not the cancer was totally removed.	If the surgeon 'got it all' the HCG level should return to normal within 6 weeks.

	You cannot use biopsies to monitor treatment.	The test is excellent for monitoring treatment progress.
	Biopsies cannot warn you of a recurrence until it is well advanced.	An increase in HCG can provide very early warning of a recurrence.

Summary

From this it is clear that the First Test Panel described here, and particularly the test for HCG in serum and urine, offers many advantages over biopsies in relation to the early detection of the start of the Cancer Process. If a return to optimum health is to be achieved by restoring systemic homeostasis the location of a potential tumour becomes of lesser importance than the earlier detection of cancer-related activity provided by the proposed tests. *Primum non nocere,* or 'first do no harm', is said to be a goal of medicine. This goal is readily achieved by the proposed tests. It is not achieved when biopsies are the method of choice for early detection.

PART III

SECOND PROPOSED TEST PANEL

A Second Test Panel is proposed. It can be used in conjunction with the First Test Panel, on its own, or after the First Test Panel. This is discussed later.

The aim of this panel is to provide further information about the faulty cellular changes that have occurred and which encourage the further development of the Cancer Process. However, it can also be used diagnostically. If, for instance, the level of HCG or PHI is raised and all the tests discussed in this Second Test Panel are normal, then it is possible that some of the other causes, indicated above, could be the cause of the raised HCG or PHI results. However, this author has had patients in whom these following tests have been abnormal when cancer was active and have returned to normal before HCG has returned to normal.

In general, however, the main aim of these tests is to establish the basis for treatment. Treatment is beyond the scope of this thesis and so the main focus of the discussion that follows is to describe the action of the substances indicated, and thus their relevance in early diagnosis.

These tests are offered by the Galkina Laboratory in Bournemouth, Dorset, UK. This laboratory also offers tests for telomerase and many other compounds that are of use in the further elucidation of the nature of cancer.

Active Proteins

PROTEIN 53 (p53)

The TP53 gene was discovered in 1979 and was the first tumour suppressor gene to be identified. It codes for protein 53, or p53. p53 is a proline-rich tumour-suppressor protein and regulates the cell cycle. The gene lies on chromosome 17. The protein is located within the cell's nucleus and binds to DNA.

The protein is activated by any damage to DNA caused by stresses, disorders or changes in cellular metabolism. When faults to DNA are detected, p53 acts in several ways. It triggers further target genes that induce cell cycle arrest so that further cells with the same faulty DNA are not produced. In this way it allows time for repairs to the damaged DNA to take place; it activates genes that in turn induce the synthesis of proteins that can accomplish this repair.

If DNA repair is not possible, p53 stimulates apoptosis of the faulty cell. Thus, p53, by regulating the cell cycle, acts to prevent mutations and hence cancer. It is thought to achieve this by binding to a p53-binding site which in turn activates the expression of further genes that act as tumour-suppressor genes and inhibit excessive growth and/or invasion. For this reason is has been referred to colloquially as 'the guardian of the genome'.

In short, p53:

*   regulates healthy cell division such that too many cell divisions and replications do not occur;
*   can stop the cell cycle at the G1/S regulation point for sufficient period of time such that the DNA can be repaired;
*   triggers the repair of faulty DNA;[315, 316]
*   triggers apoptosis of faulty cells whose DNA cannot be repaired;[317]
*   triggers senescence;
*   inhibits angiogenesis;
*   stimulates the synthesis of a second protective protein, p21.

It is involved in:

*   ageing;
*   immunity;
*   embryo implantation;
*   autophagy.

The production of p53 can be triggered by:

* genotoxic stress leading to faulty or damaged DNA;[318]
* disruption of the nucleolus;[319]
* damaged cellular membranes;
* oxidative stress;
* osmotic shock;
* heat shock;
* certain toxins;
* radiation;
* UV light;
* hypoxia, as can occur in ischemia or in rapidly growing solid tumours;[320]
* the presence of oncogenes.

The level of the p53 gene and its protein are low in healthy cells and the level of p53 is kept low by constant breakdown. Levels are frequently raised in a variety of cancer types.

Any damage to the p53 gene (TP53), such as can be caused by radiation, viruses such as HPV, and a range of chemical toxins, leads to inadequate production of p53. The same is true if only one copy of the gene is inherited. In such instances there is increased risk of the individual developing cancer. In fact, in more than half the cases of cancer, p53 is present only at very low levels or it is mutated.[321] A high level of p53 suggests the presence of cancer cells and an active p53 response. A low level suggests either the absence of cancer or the development of cancer because of inadequate p53 production.

There is an interesting interplay between p53 and vitamin D. The VDR gene codes for the receptor site for vitamin D. Vitamin D has important potential tumour-suppressive activity and this gene is up-regulated by p53.[322] Thus, it is thought that p53 may sensitise cells to the anti-proliferative actions of vitamin D3.

Mutant p53

Damage to the TP53 gene, or faulty production of p53, can lead to the formation of mutations of p53, and mutated p53 is the most commonly mutated gene in human cancers[323] and is common in a number of different human cancers. The mutant forms do not bind to the p53 binding sites and so do not trigger the tumour suppressor genes triggered by normal p53, and as a result normal tumour-suppressor activity is not stimulated and malignancy can develop. The mutated p53 builds up within the nucleus and inhibits the action of healthy p53,[324] thereby inhibiting the apoptosis that would otherwise be triggered by the damaged DNA. Thus, the presence of mutated p53 can lead to increased tumour progression and increased metastatic potential[325] and a significant negative correlation has been identified between mutated p53 expression and survival.[326]

p53 and Specific Cancers

Mutations to the TP53 are the most common mutations associated with cancer[327] and are thought to occur in about 50 per cent of people with cancer.[328] Mutated p53 gene has been detected in adrenocortical carcinoma, bladder cancer,[329] colo-rectal cancer,[330] non-small-cell lung cancer,[331, 332] osteosarcomas and more. It is reported in 20 to 40 per cent of breast cancers and is associated with larger tumours, more advanced disease and increased recurrences.[333] Its presence suggests a poor prognosis[334, 335, 336] in lymphatic cancers and non-Hodgkin's lymphomas,[337, 338] in breast cancer[339, 340] and in others, and with greater spread and increased likelihood of a recurrence following any treatment.

p53 regulates the mitochondria's electron transport chain by affecting the balance between the electron transport and glycolytic pathways. It does this via its effect on the synthesis of cytochrome c Oxidase 2 (SCO2) which regulates the COX complex, which in turn couples p53 to mitochondrial respiration and may be a contributing factor to the Warburg Effect.[341]

PROTEIN 21

Protein 21 (p21) is another protein that helps to monitor the cell cycle and, if a cell is mutated or damaged, it encourages apoptosis. p21 regulates the cell cycle of reproduction and it works with and is controlled by p53. If the level of p21 is higher than normal it suggests that cancer cells are present. If the level of p21 is lower than normal then it is probable that any cancer cells present are resisting destruction and are going to be more difficult to destroy. This is an optional test within the Second Test Panel.

PROTEIN 185 (HER2)

Human Epidermal Growth Factor Receptor 2 (HER2) or p185 is encoded by the ERBB2 gene on chromosome 17. The protein is a trans-membrane growth factor receptor involved in cell growth and development and is located on the epithelial cell membranes of most organs.

It is dangerous when over-expressed, in which case it becomes a proto-oncogene. Over-expression of this gene is found in approximately 30% of all breast cancers and is a contributing factor to the development of particularly aggressive forms of breast cancer. In addition, its presence in raised amounts suggests a poor prognosis, poor treatment response, such as decreased response to such drugs as Taxol,[342] increased risk of metastasis and poor overall outcome.[343]

p185 expression is common in NSCLC[344] and is correlated with poor clinical prognostic indicators.[345] It is also a potential contributor to cancers of the endometrium,[346] prostate,[347] colo-rectum,[348] ovaries, stomach, and the uterus.

Overall, its over-expression can lead to increased risk of tumour formation and metastasis,[349] in a variety of cancer types, and it has been suggested that p185 analysis can improve differentiation between patients with node negative, grade II, and positive or negative hormonal receptors.[350]

Some studies have shown that there is considerable overlap between patient and control values, reducing the diagnostic value of this protein.[351] However, this test becomes useful as a follow-on from the First Test Panel or as a component of the Second Test Panel if breast cancer is suspected.

p185 makes a useful early warning marker, for breast cancer in particular, as it has been detected in blood samples as early as five years prior to tumour development [Dr Olga Galkina, Galkina Laboratory, pers. comm.]. Such an early warning signal becomes invaluable as the Cancer Process can then be reversed, such that cancer need not be inevitable.

BAX, Bcl-2 AND APOPTOSIS

When cells become faulty or damaged they should self-destruct by the process of apoptosis. This is a complex process involving many genes, enzymes and related proteins including p53, BAX and Bcl-2, all of which can be readily tested for.

BAX is one of the first pro-apoptotic proteins to have been identified.[352] The nomenclature is confusing but it is also referred to as Bcl-2-associated X protein and is considered to be one of the Bcl-2 families of genes, though these are anti-apoptotic while BAX is pro-apoptotic.

BAX is present in the cytosol until apoptotic signalling triggers its insertion into the outer membrane of the mitochondria.[353] This leads to the release of pro-apoptotic factors, such as cytochrome-c, into the cytosol and triggers the activation of caspases which stimulate apoptosis.[354]

Bcl-2 (from B-cell lymphoma 2) is an apoptotic-inducing protein. Raised levels are associated with many types of cancer including breast, lung and prostate cancers, with melanomas and with lymphocytic leukemia.

The protective p53 up-regulates the production of BAX and decreases the level of Bcl-2. Conversely, mice lacking normal levels of p53 have shown decreased levels of BAX, and increased levels of Bcl-2 in several tissues.[355]

Increased levels of the Bcl-2 gene and low levels of the BAX gene have been found in people with cancer [356] and found to be useful in predicting therapeutic outcomes.[357]

Survivin and Cancer Cell Protection

The survivin gene is another, and powerful, anti-apoptotic gene, frequently associated with cancer.

The family of proteins known as IAP proteins actively inhibits apoptosis and block cell death. The group includes C-IAP1, CIAP-2, NAIP, survivin and XIAP. These proteins bind with caspase-3 and caspase-7 and interfere with or block apoptotic signalling. They are associated with fast-growing tissues, including embryo tissues and cancer tissues. They protect the cells from attack and thus reduce their level of apoptosis. In the embryo, proteins such as survivin are associated with tissues such as brain, kidneys, lungs and liver. This has an obvious and important role to play in embryonic development when rapid growth is desired, and the newly-formed cells need protection from attack or stimulation to self-destruct. Excessive apoptosis would be undesirable in a growing embryo. However, protection from apoptosis is undesirable in relation to cancer cells.

Of these proteins survivin is of particular interest and can be considered to be an oncogene. There are at least four forms of it, Survivin, Survivin-2B, Survivin-Dekta-Ex-3 and Survivin-3B.

Survivin has many functions. It protects cells, inhibits apoptosis, and regulates the normal cell cycle, especially at the mitotic process stage. These functions favour the maintenance of normal healthy tissues but are undesirable traits in cancer cells. Many studies on clinical specimens have shown that survivin gene expression is frequently increased in human cancers and is associated with resistance to chemical or radiation therapy. It indicates a poor prognosis. Conversely, it is reported that survivin inhibition, either alone or in combination with the other therapies, induces or increases apoptosis and mitotic catastrophe in tumour cells.[358]

Survivin, if present, inhibits the apoptosis that would otherwise be triggered by Fas or BAX.[359] It inhibits caspase-8 and so stops or reduces the activity of the caspase cascade near its beginning. In addition it inhibits the activation of caspase-3 and caspase-7. Survivin has also been shown to inhibit the action of cytochrome-c.

In addition to its effect on apoptosis, survivin is found in the nucleus of the cells during mitosis. It is thought to be associated with, or to contribute to, chromosome instability.

Survivin is not found associated with the fully-differentiated cells of healthy adult tissue. It has been found to be associated with transformed or cancerous cells and has been identified in all the most common cancers, including breast, prostate, colon, lung and pancreas. It's also commonly found in about 50 per cent of high-grade non-Hodgkin's lymphomas although it is not generally found in low-grade lymphomas.[360]

If the blood level survivin, or its gene, is high then it suggests both the presence of cancer cells and a higher level of difficulty in treating them. The reduction of this protein should be a major aim of any therapy programme, complementary, alternative, metabolic (CAM) or medical, drug, surgery (MDS). Once this apoptotic-blocking protein is removed, cancer cells become much more vulnerable to apoptosis.[361]

Masatsugu Ueda, et al[362] investigated survivin protein production and its gene expression and concluded that increased levels of both survivin and several matrix metalloproteinases (MMPases, see below) may work together to contribute to survival and invasion of endometriosis. Similar conclusions may be appropriate in relation to a variety of cancers. Detection of survivin or its associated gene may provide an early biomarker of aggressive tumour behaviour before the appearance of tissue abnormalities.[363]

p53 protein has been shown to reduce the cell's production of survivin and to reduce the effectiveness of its anti-apoptotic action. However, if the p53 gene is mutated this beneficial effect is lost.[364] Survivin protects cancer cells from attack by many aspects of the body's immune defences that might otherwise also destroy them. If the survivin level is high then both chemotherapy and radiation treatment are likely to be a lot less effective. Ideally the survivin level should be reduced before toxic or dangerous therapies, such as chemotherapy or radiation, are applied

Not only does survivin inhibit apoptosis, but its presence can also be used to confirm a positive diagnosis of the activity of the Cancer Process, following on from the results of the First Test Panel. Several researchers, rightly, have commented that there is an urgent need for methods of predicting aggressive tumour behaviour at the earliest stages of disease, and before there is a detectable tumour. They studied survivin, as an essential regulator of cell division and apoptosis, and concluded that increased production of survivin can induce tissue changes that may stimulate tumour production. Further, they state that, "...detection of survivin or its associated gene signature may provide an early biomarker of aggressive tumour behaviour before the appearance of tissue abnormalities." [365]

VEGF and Angiogenesis

A major requirement of cancer cells is a ready source of nutrients and the factors that will stimulate both its growth and the removal of waste. For this it needs to obtain its own blood supply. Without this, tumours rarely grow to greater than 1–2 mm^3.[366]

If there is evidence of increased angiogenesis and if there are no wounds or other indications of tissue damage, including sporting strains or injuries, and hence on-going tissue repair, evidence of increased angiogenesis could add to the probability of the Cancer Process being active.

Many factors stimulate angiogenesis, such as fibroblast growth factor (FGF), vascular endothelial growth factor (VEGF) and platelet derived growth factor (PDGF). Although their roles overlap somewhat, FGF-1 is unique in stimulating the differentiation and proliferation of all cell types necessary for the production of new arteries. FGF-2 is slightly less potent. VEGF is involved in the building of new blood capillaries within a network.[367]

The new capillaries can be produced by either splitting angiogenesis or sprouting angiogenesis. In splitting angiogenesis the capillary wall grows into the capillary lumen and then divides in such a way that the single capillary divides into two. In sprouting angiogenesis, angiogenic growth factors activate the receptor sites on existing endothelial cells on blood vessels. These activated cells then release proteases that break down the basement membrane so that endothelial cells break away, move into the surrounding matrix, proliferate and form first sprouts and then entirely new capillaries that can form in gaps in the existing network and allow it to grow. VEGF is essential for sprouting angiogenesis which can encourage growth at a rate of several mm per day and is of particular interest in tumour growth and development.[368]

MMPases and Metastatic Invasions

Another group of proteins can be increased in, and help to confirm, the diagnosis of Cancer Process activity. These are the matrix metalloproteinases or MMPases.

Hanahan and Weinberg proposed six features common to cancer cells which are an essential part of their development and survival. These are self-sufficiency in growth signals, uncontrolled growth, the avoidance of growth-inhibiting signals, avoidance of apoptosis, on-going angiogenesis and metastatic potential.[369, 370] Of these the first five apply to benign tumours. Metastatic potential is an essential feature of cancer development.

A discrete and localised tumour may do relatively little harm, unless it becomes sufficiently large such that it interferes with the normal function of the surrounding tissues or organs. The real danger comes when cancer cells disperse and relocate in other tissues, via the formation of metastasis.

It is generally thought that the metastatic process starts when cells from the primary tumour break away and travel via the blood or the lymph or both. They may come to rest in lymph glands, when the process is labelled 'nodal involvement', or they may come to rest in different tissues and constitute metastatic spread. Cells from a breast tumour may, for instance, spread to the bones and create a metastatic breast tumour. The secondary metastatic tumour always carries cells that are similar to, or in some way related to, those of the primary tumour. If the cancer cells in the second location are similar to the cells in the new location, it is not metastatic breast cancer but a new primary tumour, a bone tumour, in this instance.

The accepted thinking has been that the breast cancer cells are cells of fully-differentiated breast tissue and that they have in some way become less differentiated, and thus more able to multiply, and in the process have mutated or in other ways become faulty cells capable of multiplying out of control, into fully-developed cancer cells. The evidence on which this concept is based is the similarity of the metastatic cells at the new location to the cells of the tissue from which they are alleged to have come. However, Dr John Beard, over a century ago,[371] proposed that the original breast tumour came from totipotent breast stem cells that started to differentiate into breast tissue cells but were damaged along the way, remained partially undifferentiated and become transformed trophoblastic or tumour cells, and that some of these cells have travelled to the new location. In this hypothesis these undifferentiated (potential) breast cells were never actually fully-differentiated and developed breast cells, and they did not come from a tumour at that site. It is becoming increasingly common to see references made to cancer as deriving from incorrectly differentiated adult stem cells. Dr Biava[372] writes a particularly interesting book that covers his development of the idea.

If the source is a tumour, the metastatic process has several complex steps. A tumour is generally surrounded and kept intact by a coherent layer of connective tissue. Individual cells do not simply float away from this. Although following surgery and/or if there is any damage to this connective tissue layer, metastatic spread is more likely to occur.

In the absence of surgical disruption, the would-be breakaway cancer cells have to attack the proteins that are part of the extra-cellular matrix (ECM) surrounding the cells. Only by attaching to and damaging these ECM proteins can the cancer cells escape from their original location.

The degradation of this ECM is done by matrix metalloproteinases (MMPases). These proteins are first produced as inactive proproteins which are then broken down by extra-cellular proteases to active proteins. The MMPases act on the collagen that gives much of the strength and cohesion to the extra-cellular matrix. This process is useful in the early invasive stages of pregnancy. It also occurs but is unhelpful in diseases such as arthritis and cancer.

The released cells have to break through the basement layer of the blood vessel wall to enable them to enter the bloodstream. This process requires specific enzymes. At the new location further enzymatic breakdown of the basal membrane is required to enable the cells to leave the bloodstream and enter the new tissue. There is further resistance to the arrival of these migrating cancer cells, caused by the action of metastasis-suppressor proteins. About a dozen of these have been identified; they are helpful in that they help to reduce your risk of metastasis forming, and are all different to the proteins produced by tumour-suppressor genes.[373]

METASTASIS AND MMP-2

MMP-2 is one of the matrix metalloproteinases discussed above, and one that can be tested for. It breaks down the epithelial and basal membranes of epithelial tissues and destroys the extra-cellular matrix in which the cells of the tissues are embedded. Once this matrix breaks down it is relatively easy for an initial tumour to become established. Thus, a high level of MMP-2 can not only indicate an active Cancer Process but also suggest an increased risk of metastasis.

It is possible to measure the absolute amount of MMP-2, and other MMPases, or to measure their gene expression.

MMP-2 AND ANGIOGENESIS

MMP-2 also works with VEGF in stimulating angiogenesis. It does so by breaking down the proteins that support the original blood wall cells and structures, allowing the endothelial cells to escape into the interstitial matrix, as occurs during sprouting angiogenesis. The correct level of MMP-2 activity is important. Too little would hinder the process of angiogenesis when it is needed, too much would cause excessive tissue breakdown. During or following cancer a high level of MMP-2 can be a warning of further adverse activity.[374]

Summary

Thus we have a proposed Second Test Panel consisting of:

Protein 53 gene, mutated p53 gene and p53, BAX, Bcl-2, survivin, VEGF and MMP-2.

Optional: Protein 21, p185.

Other tests are possible and available and would provide further useful information, but that goes beyond the scope of this thesis.

PART IV

CASE HISTORIES

The basis for the tests described above is the science behind them, the biochemistry and cellular physiology, as explained. The validity of the tests is not founded on the following anecdotal case histories. These case histories are given as examples of what can be done and to illustrate some of the benefits and different uses that can be made of the tests.

Although the tests have been described as consisting of two panels, in fact they are two groups of tests, and, as is clearly demonstrated below, not everyone chooses to do all the tests in either one of the panels at any one time. This is largely due to cost. Were the tests covered by insurance then it would be possible to get all of them done on every patient, plan treatment accordingly and, in all likelihood, get an improvement more rapidly and more economically than is achieved by the MDS approach.

In the event of test results that suggest an active cancer, much of the treatment involves major changes in diet and lifestyle and a significant expenditure on remedies. Inevitably, patients are not always consistent in what they do. As a result the outcomes vary and are often not linear. However, the general progression that occurred in the first two case histories amply demonstrates the value of doing the tests and the uses that can be made of the results by those wanting to follow this approach and willing to make the appropriate effort even when their disease is far advanced. Obviously a lesser commitment is required if the tests are done much earlier on, or before the full development of the Cancer Process.

It is important to recognise that some of the test results can rise during treatment. For instance, the use of substances that are designed to create tumourlysis can result in increases in the blood or urine levels of some of the adverse breakdown products. This is one of the reasons why carefully planned detoxing programmes are an essential part of any treatment plan.

Case History 1

DS had been symptom free and healthy until she experienced several mild episodes of vaginal bleeding. After gynaecological examination and various tests she had been diagnosed with metastatic squamous cell carcinoma of the cervix, grade IIb or III with a 7 x 4 cm tumour and with myometrium, parametrium and lymph node involvement. She was advised that immediate treatment was necessary to avoid urinary reflux and kidney failure. She refused the chemotherapy and radiation options but agreed to a radical hysterectomy, after which they 'hoped they had got it all'. However, post-operatively she was told that further treatment was indicated and strongly recommended, that while chemotherapy could only help a little, their findings showed that radiation treatment was absolutely essential. Without it, she was told, death would be both imminent and very painful. Her most optimistic consultant told her that, even with radiation treatment, given her age and other factors, she would be very lucky if she had eighteen months. She was adamant in her refusal to have further medical treatment, read all she could find and put herself on a self-selected improved diet and supplement programme. Later she saw me and opted for the tests I suggested in combination with naturopathic methods of endeavouring to recover her health.

The testing started, necessarily, several months after her operation. The results are shown below. By the time of testing her HCG should have returned to normal (<0.1). It had not and it seemed possible that they had not 'got it all'. Her high PHI suggested that the Cancer Process was still active in her.

Four months later, and with more extensive naturopathic or CAM treatments, her PHI returned to within normal limits but later she expressed concern at the level of HCG and elected to do some of the tests from the Second Test Panel. Her p53 was mutated; MMP-2 was high, consistent with ready metastasis; p185 was normal. VEGF was normal but her survivin gene expression was very high, suggesting that further successful treatment could be difficult until that was resolved. Her treatment plan was adjusted accordingly.

DS	Ref/Norm	Months From First Test								
		0	4	8	13	18	25	36	38	50
HCG-IRMA	**<0.1**	1.8	1.2	1.6	1.3	1.3	1.7	1.1	0.6	1.2
HCG-IMM	**<0.1**	2.6	2.0	2.2	2.1	2.3	2.3	4.9	2.9	2.7
HCG-urine								2.8	3.0	4.5
PHI	**0 – 34**	50.3	27.3	24.0	33.2	27.3	29.2	30.0	24.4	23.7
CEA	**0.0 – 3.0**	1.7	2.2						3.6	2.1
d-Lactic acid	**0.08 – 0.17**					n.d.				
l-Lactic acid	**N.D. – Tr.**			0.70		n.d.				
TM2-PK	**5.0 – 15.0**			2.6	34.82	16.40				
Telomerase	**N.D. – Tr.**			39		1.00				
Bax	**1,000 – 10,000**								1.3×10^9	
Bcl-2 G.E.	**50 – 1,500**								3.5×10^{10}	
MMP-2	**50 – 1,500**			1.1×10^5						
p21 Gene Expression	**50 – 1,000**								1.3×10^{19}	
p53 mutated	**< 10**			20.61						
p53 protein	**> 10**								104	
p53 Gene Expression	**> 1,000**								3.8×10^6	n.d.
p185	**< 6.8**			4.50						
Survivin	**10 – 1,500**			7.8×10^5					6.6×10^8	n.d.
VEGF	**3,000 – 10,000**			1,625					6.0×10^{15}	n.d.

She continued to resist heavy persuasion to have radiation treatment. Instead she followed naturopathic treatments which were modified as appropriate, based on her test results. Three years after her first test she agreed to further tests that this time included BAX and Bacl-2 for her apoptosis activity; both were high. She continued with intermittent testing and appropriate changes to her regime and by four years from the start of testing her results were essentially down to normal levels, although p53 was lower than the desirable level.

HCG figures have remained slightly high but this could be due to the post-menopausal phenomena described earlier, although it is unwise to assume this. It can also happen that these results return to normal much later than the other abnormalities.

Clearly she has outlived the expectations placed on her, of 'eighteen months at best'. Over eight years later she is in good health, her test results are good and she continues to follow the naturopathic prevention programmes outlined in both of my books *Vital Signs for Cancer* and *Cancer Concerns*, with supplement variations depending on the latest test results. It may seem like a lengthy treatment period but in all that time she has felt well, worked and lived a normal life. She had no adverse side effects of any of the treatments, other than symptoms of detoxing, and has had many other positive benefits.

Case History 2

TS, a post-menopausal female, weighing 13.5 stone with a high-intensity career lifestyle, had been vaginally bleeding heavily for six weeks. She had seen her doctor, been referred for an ultrasound scan, told there was uterine thickening at the back of the womb and led to believe it 'was probably cancer'. The first biopsy attempt led to further heavy bleeding but a sample was not achieved. To reduce the bleeding and facilitate the next attempt she was prescribed norethisterone (a form of progesterone) that is not normally advised if cancer is suspected. A month later the second biopsy was attempted, without anaesthetic and by a junior assistant. From subsequent discussions with her doctor she was uncertain as to whether or not a viable sample had been achieved; she was assured she was 'probably all clear', but that she should return for a another check-up in a few months' time. She remained unconvinced and by then had lost confidence in her medical team.

During the latter part of this time she had come to me and we had arranged for blood and urine samples to be collected and sent off for a number of tests from the Second Test Panel. While we were waiting for these results she made radical and positive changes to her diet and started on a programme of basic supplements and detoxing.

Her test results, shown below, strongly indicate the probability of a very active Cancer Process.

	Ref/norm	Months since first test											Ref change	Units
		0	2	3	5	11-15	16	22	24	27	30	34		
IRMA					2.9	2.2				1.9		1.7		
IMM					5.3	5.4				2.6		4.9		
Urine						2.1				6.4		3.7		
PHI					26.9	30.1				26.6		32.3		
CEA					1.4	0.9				1.3		0.9		
d-Lactic acid	0.08-0.17	n.d.												mg/ml plasma
l-Lactic acid	N.D. - Tr	n.d.												
Telomerase	N.D. - Tr						9.9×10^9							No of cells/mcl
TM2-PK	5.0 - 15.0	61.70	11.10	19.30	53.50		3.00							units/ml plasma
BAX G.E.	1,000-10,000 cope/mcl						2.0×10^6	388.00	44.00	137.00	n.d.	175.00	10-100 units / mcl	
BCL-2	1,000-10,000 copies						7.9×10^6	1.3×10^{59}	1.3×10^4	n.d	n.d.	n.d	< 10 units/ mcl	copies/mcl plasma
MMP-2	50 - 1,500 copies	1.3×10^{20}	1.7×10^8	10.00	6.9×10^6	1.3×10^9	19,254	2.5×10^6	n.d.		157	n.d	10-50 units /mcl	copies/mcl plasma
p21 G.E.	50-1,000	1.7×10^{23}		3.2×10^6			4.8×10^5							
p53 G.E.	>1,000					1.8×10^6	2.7×10^{11}	1.7×10^8		1.48×10^4	n.d.		18,537.00	
p53 protein	>10	2.872					40.7	39		n.d.	n.d.	0.7	0.10-1.0	
p53.mutated G.E.													n.d.	
Survivin G.E.	10 - 1,500 copies	5.6×10^{56}	1.1×10^{14}		1207	1.7×10^{32}	83,371	7,614	1.3×10^7	n.d.	n.d.	n.d	10 units/mcl	copies/mcl plasma
VEGF G.E.	3,000 - 10,000 copies	7.0×10^{14}	5.0×10^{38}	1.9×10^{11}	7.2×10^7	6.6×10^{10}	6.3×10^{19}	2.6×10^6	1.2×10^3	n.d.	n.d.	n.d	100-1,000 units/mcl	copies/ mcl plasma

Her survivin gene expression was high, so dealing with that was the first target of her regime and extensive remedies were put in place to achieve this. By the fifth month this was down to normal and, her focus moved, financially and practically, to other parameters. As a result her survivin level rose again, though not to its initial levels, and once again had to be brought under control to enable her to obtain the maximum benefit from the other protocols she had in place.

Six months from her first consultation she had lost four stone in weight and gained enormously in energy. As a result of this weight loss she was able to detect a lump on her left breast. A thermogram of the breast indicated a probable cancer, but she refused a biopsy and stuck more closely to her full recovery programme. At this time she experienced episodes of colon bleeding.

However, she continued to refuse further conventional medical interventions, including biopsies or a colonoscopy, as she was concerned about the risk of spreading any cancer that was present. She also said that, even if the results indicate malignancy, she would not agree to surgery, radiation or chemotherapy and she was much more interested in doing all she could to improve her health and correct the results we had found by natural means.

Some of the remedies she took resulted in immediate 'burning' in the breast lump, which gradually diminished, as did the lump itself, and a second thermogram showed both breasts to be clear. Her results became essentially normal, with the same caveat as for DS above. She remains slim, healthy, energetically involved in her work and, more or less, sticking to her regime.

Case History 3

RY's story was very different. A woman in her fifties, she came to see me, saying that she just didn't feel well. She had a variety of generalised symptoms; she was tired, sick, and felt generally unwell, but with nothing she could specify. She had seen her doctor several times and been told there was nothing wrong with her, to take a tonic, have a rest, or similar. For a number of reasons I wanted to rule out cancer but didn't mention the word to her. Instead I suggested the First Test Panel as a means of finding out if her cells were going anaerobic, in which case I would have a better idea of what to do. Her results confirmed my fears.

Months since first visit	**RY**	0	11	23	27
Test	**Reference**				
HCG-IRMA	**< 0.1**	3.4	3.9	3.4	
HCG-IMM	**< 0.1**	4.8	3.7	3.7	
PHI	**0 - 34**	42.7	73.7	35.2	
CEA	**0.0 - 3.0**	0.4	0.3		
TM2-PK	**5-15 units/ml**		24.9		56.7
l-lactic acid	**Trace or n.d.**		Trace		Trace
MMP-2	**50 - 1,500**				n.d.
Survivin	**10 - 1,500**		135		1.1×10^{11}
VEGF	**3,000 - 10,000**				4.0×10^{19}

I explained the significance of the results to her. Based on the figures for HCG and PHI she was probably well into the Cancer Process and I was concerned that she could have an active tumour, somewhere in her body, as yet undetected. At this time urinary HCG levels were not offered by the laboratory. It is pertinent to remember that these results do not give any indication as to location, they refer to the systemic state and that the location is of less importance to a naturopathic physician than to a medical doctor as any proposed naturopathic treatment will also be systemic, rather than tumour-focused.

RY was not convinced of the seriousness of the problem but agreed to see her doctor again. However, he made light of the results, said HCG was only relevant in cancers related to pregnancy, and told her she need not worry. Her friends reinforced this saying that if the doctor did not think the results were significant there was clearly nothing to worry about and she should not be concerned. Sadly this reduced her commitment to the treatment plan I suggested, but she did decide to follow at least part of it.

Eleven months later she repeated the First Test Panel. The results showed her PHI result to have worsened. Although she still remained unconvinced of the seriousness of the situation this did stimulate her to increase some of her treatment options, saying that at least she was feeling better as a result of what she had already been doing.

At 23 months her PHI had come down to almost within the reference range, but there was little improvement in the HCG. She had told her doctor of epigastric pain and it had been suggested to her that she may have a hiatus hernia. When I next contacted her she was still feeling unwell and agreed to some more tests, notably focusing on the Second Test Panel. Although MMP-2 was normal, suggesting a relatively low risk of metastasis, which was borne out by future events, her survivin gene expression had gone from normal to very high and VEGF gene expression was also high. Both were of great concern.

I advised her strongly to see her doctor again and say she was concerned about cancer and wanted to explore this possibility. She came back from that saying she had had a mammogram and pap smear and they were both normal and she was 'fine'.

Three months later she told me it had taken her an hour to eat a meal. I again advised her to see a doctor and this time to ask for a stomach scan. In this she was unsuccessful. She was told that she had an acid stomach and had been given an antacid. I finally persuaded her to go straight back and insist on a scan which she was at last able to organise. It showed a large stomach tumour. No metastatic spread was detected. Unfortunately, by this time, swallowing was difficult and taking any remedy in capsule or tablet form had become impossible. She did her best with liquid and powdered supplements, but at this late stage the treatments she could take were insufficient and she did not respond to any medical treatment. She died just over a year later.

This case history exemplifies the frustrations that can occur when patients are (a) reluctant to do the tests because of the costs, and because they are afraid to know the results; and (b) are too easily persuaded to ignore these warnings, preferring to believe that things are not as bad as they seem when told so by someone, even their doctor, who does not understand this work.

Case History 4

PD, a male in his sixties, used the First Test Panel for a different purpose. He had had major surgery after being diagnosed with a large prostate tumour. Recognising the uncertainty of the PSA test and its specificity for cancer he wanted some other markers with which he could monitor his progress. He did PSA tests every few months, and every time they rose at all it was suggested that he should consider various drug protocols. He was reluctant to agree to this.

He did part of the First Test Panel twice, five and eight years after diagnosis and his results, shown below, reassured him that he was almost certainly in remission. It would be better had the PHI not increased, as any increase after a diagnosis of cancer can be an early warning sign of a possible recurrence. However, the second set of results was obtained over two years ago and he remains in good health ten years after his initial diagnosis.

PD			
Test	Reference		3 Years later
HCG-IRMA	< 0.1	0.00	0.00
HCG-IMM	< 0.1	0.00	0.00
PHI	0 - 34	24	35.5
CEA	0.0 - 3.0	1.3	1.7

Case History 5

OJ's story shows the wisdom of not relying on a single test, or even the First Test Panel alone if even one result is abnormal. She presented with a history of biopsy-proven breast cancer followed by a mastectomy and chemotherapy to which she had reacted badly and which was stopped by her doctors. Radiation was suggested but she refused it. Eight years later she was diagnosed with extensive metastasis and a diagnosis of Stage IV. Following significant naturopath treatments over the next two years her CA markers normalised, but she then found a lump in her remaining breast.

She adamantly refused conventional medical treatment and came to me for, in her mind, palliative care. Her first set of results showed no HCG but a very high PHI, of over 70. This latter was supported by symptoms such as extreme fatigue. Because of the raised PHI we then did the Second Test Panel to learn more and found raised, supportive p53 but also raised harmful, mutated p53. In addition, some of the other markers in the profile were abnormal and had to be worked on. Reliance on the First Test Panel alone might have led to a more sanguine diagnosis which would have been unsafe.

Case History 6:

Another discussion is pertinent.

MB attended one of my talks in which I discussed the importance of the tests described in this thesis, particularly the First Test Panel. When she spoke to me afterwards she said she would never do such tests as she would be terrified of the results; if they were abnormal, she did not think she could face the medical treatments. I discussed with her the naturopathic treatments and the evidence that much could be done to reverse the Cancer Process by natural means, particularly when or if it is detected at the very early stage, as these tests can do. Once she fully understood this she said she would be delighted to do at least the First Test Panel, and could well see the point of doing so.

In summary these are several people who have made use of or responded to the concepts described in this thesis in very different ways. One had a known cancer with nodal and metastatic spread, had surgery but refused further medical treatment, did the tests and went on a recovery protocol dictated by these test results, particularly those of the Second Test Panel.

A second person had urine, blood and thermogram tests that strongly indicated an active Cancer Process, did the tests discussed here, went on recovery protocols indicated by these tests and now has clear test results.

The health of both these women has improved and they now, several years later, have excellent test results. In the case of DS, specified longevity has been greatly increased.

The third woman did some of both the First and Second Test Panels. Her results strongly indicated cancer; she largely ignored this warning, and progressed to a large tumour mass and died soon after.

OJ's case illustrates the benefit of doing both test panels. PD used the results from the First Test Panel to resist his specialist's suggestion of drug treatments and has outlived the expectation he was given.

Finally, there is a woman who eventually recognised the benefit of doing these tests and the fact that even adverse results need not lead to painful, toxic or unpleasant therapies.

SUMMARY

It is proposed that cancer is a process. This process starts long before a tumour is formed or can be detected. The results of analysis of blood and urine samples can indicate the Cancer Process, arguably after only about six weeks of development.

The aim of this thesis has been to show that there is a First Test Panel or group of tests that, taken together, have a high probability of detecting very early changes indicative of this Cancer Process, and of doing so long before a detectable tumour has formed. There is also a second group of tests that can provide important information as to the nature of the adverse biochemical and cellular errors that are occurring and this information can be used to inform the appropriate treatment protocol.

Because this panel detects the very early stages of the Cancer Process, therapeutic changes can be implemented at a much earlier stage, and with a far better probability of success, than if the diagnosis is delayed until a tumour can be detected.

The initial test was for human chorionic gonadotropin (HCG). In the 1950s, through the work of Dr Manuel Navarro and Dr Howard Beard, a Yale trained biologist and chemistry professor, the Anthrone Colour Test, done on a urine sample, was used to detect the possible presence of HCG.[375] However, this test did not discriminate between the alpha and beta sub-units and only indicated total HCG-like components. It was a start, but has been superseded as an early warning test by the combination of urine and serum tests for HCG, by different analytical techniques.

HCG has been shown to be associated with a very wide range of cancer types. The tests required to detect cancer at the early stages of cancer have to be very sensitive and as this sensitivity improves even further it is possible that HCG will be found to be more closely associated with an increasing number of cancer types. It is also possible that, as the tests improve, a greater proportion of people with any type of cancer will be found to be HCG positive.

False positives are almost certainly rare. If HCG is raised in someone without an existing diagnosis of cancer it is more likely to be a true result and an early warning sign than a false positive. It may be important to consider making allowance for raised levels in post-menopausal women and older men, but care must be taken that true positives are not ignored by incorrectly attributing them to menopausal or age-related levels rather than cancer.

The first panel is extended by the addition of phosphohexose isomerase (PHI), an enzyme in the cytosol's Embden-Meyerhof pathway, indicative of increased activity of that pathway and increased anaerobic activity of the cells. It is postulated that this increase in anaerobic activity is accompanied by, and indicative of, decreased mitochondrial function, which in turn, according to Dr Otto Warburg in 1933 and many others since, and in association with reduced cellular oxygen, is the ultimate cause of cancer. Increased anaerobic function is associated with increased risk of cancer.

These four tests, three for HCG and one for PHI are, arguably, the foundation of the First Test Panel. However, it is suggested that, to reduce the risk of false negative results, other tests be added and that they include tests for l-lactic acid, carcino embryonic antigen (CEA), telomerase and, optionally, tumour marker 2 pyruvate kinase (TM2-PK).

Not only does this panel, if the test results are positive (high), indicate the possibility of the activity of the Cancer Process, it also gives some indications as to possible treatment directions. These can include improving mitochondrial function and blood glucose management, and the removal of l-lactic acid.

It is hoped that treatment plans would be compatible with the health of the body and follow the lines of CAM therapies. These therapies are helpful generally as well as specifically and, as such, any false positive results, if treated by CAM methods, while being worrying to the individual, could still provide benefit. Medical, invasive and toxic treatments should not be implemented on the basis of these tests alone.

False negatives are possible and this must be considered during follow-up clinical discussions and diagnosis. When the full First Test Panel is utilised it provides a useful, whole body, detection test for the possible start of the Cancer Process.

Any false negatives are of more concern and the detection of the Cancer Process would then be delayed, as would corrective measures. The risk of false negatives is of greater concern than the risk of false positives. It is for this reason that several tests have been proposed, in an extensive panel, with a greater possibility of avoiding false negatives.

If the results from the First Test Panel are ambiguous, and further testing is wanted, a Second Test Panel is suggested. This Second Test Panel can provide further corroboration of a positive indication of the cancer. Alternatively it can help to suggest that the results of the first test may have other explanations than cancer. Importantly, it gives many further indications as to the direction a treatment protocol should take.

This Second Test Panel includes testing for the proteins p53, p21 (optional), p185, for BAX and Bcl-2, which impact on apoptosis, for the survivin gene, which codes for a protein that protects cancer cells, for the matrix metalloproteinases such as MMP-2, and for angiogenesis stimulators such as VEGF.

Correction procedures are covered in my other books in this series and are beyond the remit of this thesis but should be aimed at restoring the body to normal function by thorough and probably radical, dietary, lifestyle and nutrient changes, in conjunction with a wide variety of plant-derived and related nutrients and natural remedies and therapies. These can, when properly put in place, restore the cells to full, aerobic mitochondrial function, and the body to greater health. These strategies can be considered to be reversing the Cancer Process, if this has started. If it has not, and the results are indeed false positives, the corrections will in any case improve the overall health of the individual and provide a good chance that the individual avoids a possible future occurrence of cancer, as well as helping to prevent other degenerative diseases.

A concept outlined in Section I bears repetition here. There is, in general, an unwillingness on the part of the medical profession to run screening tests on a wide scale, especially those aimed at prevention rather than treatment. However, it is suggested here that if this panel of tests was made widely available, and if individuals were willing to make the indicated and necessary changes to their diet and lifestyle, a significant proportion of cases of cancer and of early deaths from cancer, could be avoided. This could also result in a great reduction to the overall healthcare expenditure.

APPENDIX 1

Laboratories

Appreciation is due to the directors of the first two laboratories for the help they have given me and for offering the tests indicated so that many people can benefit from their results.

American Metabolic Laboratories,
Director: Dr Schandl
Address: 1818 Sheriden Street, Suite 102, Hollywood, Florida FL 33020, USA
www.caprofile.net. Email: info@caprofile.net. (+1) 954-929-4814

Tests: HCG, PHI, CEA, telomerase (in development).

The Galkina Laboratory Limited
Director: Dr Galkina
Address: 681 Wimbourne Road, Bournemouth, Dorset, BH9 2AT, UK
www.neuro-lab.com. Email:drtaylor@thegalkinalab.co.uk. T: 44-1202-510910

Tests: p53, mutated and wild, p21, BAX, Bcl-2, MMP-2, survivin, telomerase, VEGF.

Genova Diagnostics
Address: 63 Zillicoa Street, Asheville, NC 28801, USA
Telephone: 800-522-4762
www.gdx. Email via website. T: (+1) 800-522-4762: (+1)-828-253-0621

Tests: Lactic acid, and many other general but useful tests.

BioLab Medical Unit
Address: The Stone House, 9 Weymouth Street, London W1W 6DB, UK
Telephone: (+44) 020-7636-5959
Tests: Many useful nutritional and related tests, including tests for toxins.

APPENDIX II

GLOSSARY

Activin	A protein complex that increases synthesis of FSH and secretin, regulates the menstrual cycle and plays a role in cell proliferation and differentiation.
Adenocarcinoma	Cancer of epithelial tissue originating in glandular tissue.
Abbott Diagnostics AxSym HCGβ	Used in pregnancy testing.
Aneuploidy	Abnormal number of chromosomes, which can lead to genetic disorders and birth defects.
Autocrine signalling	Signalling in which a cell secretes an autocrine agent (a hormone or chemical messenger) that binds to autocrine receptors on the same cell, leading to changes within the cell.
CA 15-3	Breast (late).
CA 19-9	Bladder, colo-rectal (late), pancreas (follow-up), stomach.
CA 27-29	Breast (late).
CA 72-4	Stomach.
CA 125	Bladder, ovarian.
Caspases	Cysteine-aspartate-proteases, involved in apoptosis, necrosis and inflammation.
CD44	Protein. Receptor for hyaluronic acid. Interacts with MMPases. Variations occur in some cancers – breast and prostate stem cells, endometrial, head and neck cancers.
C-myc	Proto-oncogene. When switched on it stimulates telomerase.
Cytokine	Small, signalling proteins or glycoproteins, intercellular communication. E.g. Interleukins, interferons. Review.[376]
Endocrine signalling	Signalling caused by a hormone, usually from a gland, that acts systemically on selected target tissues throughout the body.

Epitopes The parts of the antigen recognised by the immune system.

ERK Extracellular signalling-regulated kinases. Activation of mitochondrial ERK increases resistance to apoptosis.

Fas-ligand Membrane protein in the TNF family. Its binding to receptors induces apoptosis.

Flow cytometry Laser based. Suspends cells in a fluid and passes them by electronic detection equipment. Used in health diagnostics especially blood cancers.

FSH Follicle stimulating hormone.

Glucagonoma A very rare tumour of the islet cells of the pancreas, which leads to an excess blood glucagon. Usually malignant with high blood sugar level (BSL) and thirst.

HER2 Human Epidermal Growth Factor, a protein found on the surface of breast cells. High levels can stimulate cell reproduction and the growth of breast cancers.

Hyaluronic acid Part of the extra-cellular matrix (ECM). Increases viscosity of extra-cellular fluid. Contributes to tumour growth via interaction with CD44 receptors (increases EC-degrading enzymes). Aids metastasis by degrading ECM. Part of wound healing.

Inhibin A secreted protein with tumour-suppressor activity, it down-regulates FSH synthesis and inhibits FSH secretion.

Intercellular Between cells.

Intracellular Inside the cell.

Monoclonal antibody tests Monoclonal specific antibodies that are the same because they are made by identical immune cells that are all clones of a unique parent cell.

MYC (c-MYC) A regulatory gene, up-regulates many genes involved in cell proliferation, can become an oncogene when mutated.

Neurotrophic factors Assist the survival of neurons by inhibiting apoptosis.

Neurotrophins A family of proteins involved in the development, function and survival of neurons. They induce progenitor cells to form neurons.

NF-κB **cells**	Nuclear-factor-kappa-light chain enhancer of B complex. Incorrect regulation of it is linked to cancer and inflammation. It controls transcription of DNA and cell proliferation. Blocking it reduces cancer cell proliferation,[377] it enhances tumour cell sensitivity to apoptosis and senescence and promotes Fas-mediated apoptosis.[378]
NK cells	A type of cytotoxic granular lymphocyte. Critical to innate immunity. Fast response to viruses, cancer cells.
Non-small-cell lung cancer	Relatively resistant to chemotherapy.
NGF	Nerve growth factor, angiogenic.
Nucleoside	Sugar + base + ribose.
Nucleotides	Sugar + base + ribose + 1-3 phosphate groups.
PAP	Peroxidase-antiperoxidase technique for HCG – less sensitive.
Paracrine signalling	Signalling in which a cell secretes an agent near to the target (receptor) cell.
Paraneoplastic	Not cancer but a disease that is a consequence of cancer.
Platelet-derived growth factor beta	A protein that regulates cell growth and division, and angiogenesis. A potent mitogen.
pRb	Retinoblastoma protein – tumour suppressor protein. Blocks inappropriate activity of the cell cycle.
PUMA p53	Up-regulated Modulator of Apoptosis.
Purines	Adenine, guanine.
Pyramidines	Cytosine, thymine (uracil in RNA).
Ras genes	Carry extra-cellular messages to the nucleus. Code for cell growth, differentiation and survival. When mutated allow excessive growth. The most common form of mutation in cancer.
Sarcolemma	The cell membrane of muscle cells.
Small-cell lung cancer	Strongly associated with smoking.
Squamous cell carcinoma	Cancer of squamous epithelial cells and cavity linings.
TGF-beta	Transforming Growth Factor-beta. Protein. Controls cell proliferation and differentiation,

affects immune function, stimulates p21 and apoptosis, stops the cell cycle at G1 stage, converts effector T-cells to suppressor T-cells thus turning off the inflammatory response. Mutated in cancer, leading to fibroblast proliferation, immune suppression, angiogenesis and invasion.

TNFs Tumour necrosis factors, proapoptotic cytokines.

TPA 12-O-tetra-decanoyl-phorbol-13-acetate.

TRAIL TNF-related apoptosis-inducing ligand. A cytokine.

Transitional cell carcinoma (TCC) Also called urothelial cell carcinoma. Usually occurs in the urinary system and accessory organs and arises from the transitional epithelium lining the inner surface of these hollow organs.

TRK Tyrosine receptor kinase, stimulates cell differentiation.

WNT A proto oncogene, involved in embryo development and increased rate of cell reproduction.

Xenobiotic A chemical found in an organism that is not normally produced or present in it.

XIAP X-linked inhibitor of apoptosis protein.

REFERENCES

[1] Michael A. Kiebish et al., *Cardiolipin and electron transport chain abnormalities in mouse brain tumour mitochondria: lipidomic evidence supporting the Warburg theory of cancer.* Journal of Lipid Research, 2008; 49(12): 2545–2556.

[2] Kang, S.H., Bang, Y.J., Im, Y.H., Yang, H.K., Lee, D.A., Lee, H.Y., Lee, H.S., Kim, N.K., Kim, S.J., *Transcriptional repression of the transforming growth factor-beta type I receptor gene by DNA methylation results in the development of TGF-beta resistance in human gastric cancer.* Oncogene 1999; 18(51): 7280–7286

[3] J. Masquelier with B. Schwitters, *OPC in Practice. The French paradox explained.* 1993

[4] B. Barnes, *Hypothyroidism: The Unsuspected Illness.* Fitzhenry and Whiteside Limited, 1976

[5] Schöler, Hans R., *The Potential of Stem Cells: An Inventory.* In Nikolaus Knoepffler, Dagmar Schipanski, and Stefan Lorenz Sorgner. 2007; *Humanbiotechnology as Social Challenge.* Ashgate Publishing. p. 28. ISBN: 978-0-7546-5755-2.

[6] S. Thorlacius, S. Sigurdsson, H. Bjarnadottir, G. Olafsdottir, J.G. Jonasson, L. Tryggvadottir, H. Tulinius, J.E. Eyfjörd, *Study of a single BRCA2 mutation with high carrier frequency in a small population.* Am. J. Hum. Genetics 1997; 60(5): 1079–1084

[7] Warburg, O., *On the origin of cancer cells.* Science 1956; 123(3191): 309–14

[8] Warburg, O., *On the origin of cancer cells.* Science 1956; 123(3191): 309–14

[9] Otto Warburg, *The Prime Cause and Prevention of Cancer.* Lecture to Nobel Laureates, 1966, June 30

[10] http://healingtools.tripod.com/primecause1.html

[11] José M. Cuezva, Maryla Krajewska, Miguel López de Heredia, Stanislaw Krajewski, Gema Santamaría, Hoguen Kim, Juan M. Zapata, Hiroyuki Marusawa, Margarita Chamorro and John C. Reed, *The bioenergetic signature of cancer, a marker of tumour progression.* Cancer Research 2002; 62: 6674–6681

[12] John, A.P., *Dysfunctional mitochondria, not oxygen insufficiency, cause cancer cells to produce inordinate amounts of lactic acid: the impact of this on the treatment of cancer.* Med. Hypothesis 2001; 57(4): 429–432

[13] Muniswamy Madesh, Lakshmi Bhaskar and K.A. Balasubramanian, *Enterocyte viability and mitochondrial function after graded intestinal ischemia and reperfusion in rats.* Mol. and Cell Biochem. 1997; 167(1-2): 81–87

[14] Robert A. Gatenby and Robert J. Gillies, *Why do cancers have high aerobic glycolysis?* Nature Reviews Cancer 2004; 4: 891–899

[15] Seyfried, T. N., *Cancer as a metabolic disease.* Wiley, 2012

[16] Hanahan, D., Weinberg, R.A., *The hallmarks of cancer.* Cell 2000; 100: 57–70

[17] Hanahan, D., Weinberg, R.A., *Hallmarks of cancer: the next generation.* Cell 2011; 144(5): 646–74

[18] P. Biava, *Cancer and the Search for Lost Meaning.* North Atlantic Books, 2009

[19] Preetha Anand, Ajaikumar B. Kunnumakara, Chitra Sundaram, Kuzhuvelil B. Harikumar, Sheeja T. Tharakan, Oiki S. Lai, Bokyung Sung and Bharat B. Aggarwal, *Cancer is a Preventable Disease that Requires Major Lifestyle Changes.* Pharm. Res. 2008; 25(9): 2097–2116

[20] Parkin, D.M., *The fraction of cancer attributable to lifestyle and environmental factors in the UK in 2010.* Br. J. Cancer 2011; 105(S2): Si–S81

[21] Morgan, G., Ward, R., Barton, M., *The contribution of cytotoxic chemotherapy to 5-year survival in adult malignancies.* Clin. Oncol. (R. Coll. Radiol.) 2004; 16: 549–560

[22] Bria, E., Gralla, R.J., Raftopoulos, H., Cuppone, F., Milella, M., Sperduti, I. et al., *Magnitude of benefit of adjuvant chemotherapy for non-small cell lung cancer: meta-analysis of randomized clinical trials.* Lung Cancer 2009; 63: 50–57

[23] Biava, Pier Mario, 2009. *Cancer and the Search for Lost Meaning.* ISBN: 978-1-55643-778-6

[24] Lichtenstein, P., Holm, N. et al., *Environmental and heritable factors in the causation of cancer.* NEJM; 343: 78–85

[25] Fryda, Dr Waltrout, 1987. *Adrenalin deficiency as the cause of cancer formation.* 2000. 4th Edition, Kunst and Alltag, Munich ISBN: 3-88410-079-3

[26] Fryda, Dr Waltraut, *Diagnosis: Cancer.* ISBN: 978-1-59926-897-2, available from www.Xlibris.com

[27] Warburg, O., *On the origin of cancer cells.* Science 1956; 123: 309–14

[28] Otto Warburg, *The Prime Cause and Prevention of Cancer.* Lecture to Nobel Laureates, 1966, June 30

[29] Fryda, Dr Waltrout, 1987, *Adrenalin deficiency as the cause of cancer formation.* 4th Edition, Kunst and Alltag, Munich ISBN: 3-88410-079-3

[30] Moritz, A., *Cancer Is Not a Disease, It's a Survival Mechanism.* 2005 (3rd edition), USA, Ener-chi Wellness Press

[31] Otto Warburg, *The Prime Cause and Prevention of Cancer.* Lecture to Nobel Laureates, 1966, June 30

[32] http://healingtools.tripod.com/primecause1.html

33   José M. Cuezva, Maryla Krajewska, Miguel López de Heredia, Stanislaw Krajewski, Gema Santamaría, Hoguen Kim, Juan M. Zapata, Hiroyuki Marusawa, Margarita Chamorro and John C. Reed, *The bioenergetic signature of cancer, a marker of tumour progression.* Cancer Research 2002; 62: 6674–6681

34   Koonin, E.V., *The two empires and the three domains of life in the postgenomic age.* Nature Education 2020; 3(9): 27

35   Habib, S.J.H., *Biogenesis and function of mitochondrial outer membrane proteins.* 2009, dissertation, Ludwig-Maximilians University of Munich

36   P. Biava., *Cancer and the Search for Lost Meaning.* North Atlantic Books, 2009

37   Preetha Anand, Ajaikumar B. Kunnumakara, Chitra Sundaram, Kuzhuvelil B. Harikumar, Sheeja T. Tharakan, Oiki S. Lai, Bokyung Sung, and Bharat B. Aggarwal, *Cancer is a Preventable Disease that Requires Major Lifestyle Changes.* Pharm. Res., 2008; 25(9): 2097–2116

38   Hanahan, D., Weinberg, R.A., *The hallmarks of cancer.* Cell 2000; 100: 57–70

39   Hanahan, D., Weinberg, R.A., *Hallmarks of cancer: the next generation.* Cell 2011; 144(5): 646–74

40   Klein, C.A., *The Metastasis Cascade.* Science 2008; 321(5897): 1785–1787

41   E.K. Schandl, *The Cancer Profile and its Clinical Application.* Townsend Letter, 2010 Aug/Sept

42   Kiberstis, P.A., *Medicine Rethinking Cancer Metastasis.* Science Signalling 2008; 1(39): 341

43   Preetha Anand, Ajaikumar B. Kunnumakara, Chitra Sundaram, Kuzhuvelil B. Harikumar, Sheeja T. Tharakan, Oiki S. Lai, Bokyung Sung, and Bharat B. Aggarwal, *Cancer is a Preventable Disease that Requires Major Lifestyle Changes.* Pharm. Res. 2008; 25(9): 2097–2116

44   Allin, K.H., Nordestgaard, B.G., *Elevated C-reactive protein in the diagnosis, prognosis, and cause of cancer.* Crit. Rev. Clin. Lab. Sci. 2011; 48(4): 155–70

45   Thomas P. Erlinger, Elizabeth A. Platz, Nader Rifai, Kathy J. Helzlsouer, *C-Reactive Protein and the Risk of Incident Colorectal Cancer.* JAMA. 2004; 291(5): 585–590

46   Claire Siemes, Loes E. Visser, Jan-Willem W. Coebergh, Ted A.W. Splinter, Jacqueline C.M. Witteman, André G. Uitterlinden, Albert Hofman, Huibert A.P. Pols, Bruno H.Ch. Stricker, *C-Reactive Protein Levels, Variation in the C-Reactive Protein Gene, and Cancer Risk: The Rotterdam Study.* J. Clin. Oncol. 2006; 24(33): 5216–5222

47   Nozoe T., Matsumata T., Kitamura M., Sugimachi K., *Significance of preoperative elevation of serum C-reactive protein as an indicator for prognosis in colorectal cancer.* American Journal of Surgery 1998; 176(4): 335–338

[48] Rink, L., Kirchner, H., *Recent progress in the tumour necrosis factor-alpha field.* Int. Arch. Allergy Immunol. 1996; 111(3): 199–209

[49] Theodore D.K. Chung, Jianqing J. Yu, Michael T. Spiotto, Michelle Bartkowski, Jonathan W. Simons, *Characterization of the role of IL-6 in the progression of prostate cancer.* Prostate 1999; 38(3): 199–207

[50] Martín, F., Santolaria, F., Batista, N., Milena, A., González-Reimers, E., Brito, M.J., Oramas, J., *Cytokine levels (IL-6 and IFN-gamma), acute phase response and nutritional status as prognostic factors in lung cancer.* Cytokine 1999; 11(1): 80–86

[51] Maie A.R. St. John, Yang Li, Xiaofeng Zhou, Paul Denny, Chih-Ming Ho, Carlo Montemagno, Wenyuan Shi, Fengxia Qi, Benjamin Wu, Uttam Sinha, Richard Jordan, Lawrence Wolinsky, No-Hee Park, Honghu Liu, Elliot Abemayor, David T.W. Wong, *Interleukin 6 and Interleukin 8 as Potential Biomarkers for Oral Cavity and Oropharyngeal Squamous Cell Carcinoma.* Arch. Otolaryngology Head Neck Surg. 2004; 130: 929–93

[52] Yuan, A., Chen, J.J., Yao, P.L., Yang, P.C., *The role of interleukin-8 in cancer cells and microenvironment interaction.* Front Biosci. 2005; 10: 853–65

[53] http://www.cancerresearchuk.org/cancer-info/cancerstats/types/breast/incidence/uk-breast-cancer-incidence-statistics

[54] www.cancer.org/Treatment/UnderstandingYourDiagnosis/ExamsandTestDescriptions/TumourMarkers/tumour-markers-common-ca-and-t-m

[55] Lapthorn, A.J., Harris, D.C., Littlejohn, A., Lustbader, J.W., Canfield, R.E., Machin, K.J., Morgan, .FJ., Isaacs, N.W., *Crystal structure of human chorionic gonadotropin.* Nature 1984; 369 (6480): 455–61

[56] Pierce, J.G. and Parsons, T.F., *Glycoprotein hormones: structure and function.* Annual Rev. Biochem. 1981; 50: 465

[57] Pierce, J.G. and Parsons, T.F., *Glycoprotein hormones: structure and function.* Annual Rev. Biochem. 1981; 50: 465–495

[58] Mann, K. and Karl, H.J., *Molecular heterogeneity of human chorionic gonadotropin and its sub-units in testicular cancer.* Cancer 1983; 52: 654–660

[59] Elliott, M.M., Kardana, A., Lustbader, J.W. and Cole, L.A., *Carbohydrate and peptide structure of the alpha- and beta-sub-units of human chorionic gonadotropin from normal and aberrant pregnancy and choriocarcinoma.* Endocrine 1997; 7: 15–32

[60] Lapthorn, A.J., Harris, D.C., Littlejohn, A., Lustbader, J.W., Canfield, R.E., Machin, K.J., Morgan, F.J., Isaacs, N.W., *Crystal structure of human chorionic gonadotropin.* Nature 1994; 369(6480): 455–61

[61] Gillott, D.J., Iles, R.K. and Chard, T., *The effects of beta-human chorionic gonadotrophin on the in vitro growth of bladder cancer cell lines.* Br. J. Cancer 1996; 73: 323–326

[62] Butler, S.A., Staite, E.M. and Iles, R.K., *Reduction of bladder cancer cell growth in response to HCGbeta CTP37 vaccinated mouse serum.* Oncol. Res. 2003; 14: 93–100

[63] Kovalevskaya, G., Genbacev, O., Fisher, S.J., Caceres, E. and O'Connor, J.F., *Trophoblast origin of HCG isoforms: cytotrophoblasts are the primary source of choriocarcinoma-like HCG.* Mol. Cell Endocrinol. 2002; 194: 147–155

[64] Filicori, M., Fazleabas, A.T., Huhtaniemi, I., Licht, P., Rao, Ch.V., Tesarik, J. and Zygmunt, M., *Novel concepts of human chorionic gonadotropin: reproductive system interactions and potential in the management of infertility.* Fertil. Steril. 2005; 84: 275–284

[65] Kayisli, U., Selam, B., Guzeloglu-Kayisli, O., Demir, R., Arici, A., *Human chorionic gonadotropin contributes to maternal immunotolerance and endometrial apoptosis by regulating Fas-Fas ligand system.* J. Immunol. 2003; 171(5): 2305–13

[66] Askling, J., Erlandsson, G., Kaijser, M., Akre, O., Ekbom, A., *Sickness in pregnancy and sex of child.* Lancet 1999; 354(9195): 2053

[67] Michels, K.B., Xue, F., Colditz, G.A., Willett, W.C., Induced and spontaneous abortion and incidence of breast cancer among *young women: a prospective cohort study.* Arch. Intern. Med. 2007; 167 (8): 814–20

[68] *Recherches dur le Traitement du Cancer, etc.* Paris. Editoral Archiv fuer pathologische Anatomie und Physiologie und fuer klinische Medizin 1829; 8(1855): 23

[69] Durante, F., *Nesso fisio-pathologico tra la struttura dei nei materni e la genesi di alcuni tumouri maligni.* Arch. Memor. Observ. Chir. Pract. 1874; 11: 217–26

[70] Beard, J., *The enzyme treatment of cancer and its scientific basis.* First published 1911, Republished 2010, New Spring Press

[71] Recamier, J.C.A., *Recherches sur le traitement du cancer: par la compression methodique simple ou combinee, et sur l'histoire general de la meme maladie.* 1829; 2

[72] Remark, R., *Ein beitrag zur entwickelungsgeschichte der citric acidhaften geschwulste.* Deut. Klin. 1854; 6: 70–174

[73] Durante, F., *Nesso fisio-pathologico tra la struttura dei nei materni e la genesi di alcuni tumouri maligni.* Arch. Memori eed Osservazioni di chirugia practica 1874; 11: 217–226

[74] Cohnheim, J., *Congenitales, quergestreiftes muskelsarkon der nireren.* Virchows Arch. 1875; 65: 64

[75] Stewart Sell. *Alpha-fetoprotein (AFP), stem cells, and cancer: how study of the production of AFP during chemical hepatocarcinogenesis led to reaffirmation of the stem cell theory of cancer.* Tumour Biol. 2008; 29(3): 161–180

76 http://www.scienceblog.com/cms/scientists_find_stem_cells_in_human_breast_cancer

77 Fishman, W.H., Sell, S., *Onco-developmental gene expression.* NY Acad. Press Inc.; 1976: 1–788

78 Pierce, G.B., Shikes, R., Fink, L.M., *Cancer: a problem of developmental biology.* Engelweed Cliffs, NJ, Prentice Hall Inc.; 1978: 1–242

79 Canfield, R.E., Ross, G.T., *A new reference preparation of human chorionic gonadotrophin and its sub-units.* Bulletin of the World Health Organization 1976; 54(4): 463–472

80 Waddell, Rebecca Smith (2006), *Home Pregnancy Test HCG Levels and FAQ.* http://www.fertilityplus.org/faq/hpt.html

81 http://www.americanpregnancy.org/duringpregnancy/HCGlevels.html

82 Schandl, E.K., *The cancer profile and its clinical applications.* Townsend Newsletter 2010; Aug-Sept

83 Jennifer A. Snyder, Shannon Haymond, Curtis A. Parvin, Ann M. Gronowski, David G. Grenache, *Diagnostic Considerations in the Measurement of Human Chorionic Gonadotropin in Aging Women.* Clinical Chemistry, 2005; 51(10): 1830–1835

84 Stenman, U.H., Alfthan, H. and Hotakainen, K., *Human chorionic gonadotropin in cancer.* Clin. Biochem. 2004; 37: 549–561

85 Seckl, M.J., Sebire, N.J., Berkowitz, R.S., *Gestational trophoblastic disease.* Lancet 2001; 376 (9742): 717–29

86 Lurain, J.R., *Gestational trophoblastic disease I: epidemiology, pathology, clinical presentation and diagnosis of gestational trophoblastic disease, and management of hydatidiform mole.* Am. J. Obstet. Gynecol. 2019; 203 (6): 531–9

87 http://cancer.stanford.edu/information/cancerDiagnosis

88 Stenman, U.H., Alfthan, H., Hotakainen, K., *Human Chorionic Gonadotropin in Cancer.* Clinical Biochemistry 2004; 37: 549–561

89 McManus, L.M., Naughton, N.A., Martinex, H.A.A., *Human chorionic gonadotropin in human neoplastic cells.* Cancer Res. 1976; 36: 3476

90 Braunstein, G.D., Vaitukaitis, J.L., Carbone, P.P. and Ross, G.T., *Ectopic production of human chorionic gonadotrophin by neoplasms.* Ann. Intern. Med. 1973; 78: 39–45

91 Tormey, D.C., Waalkes, T.P., Simon, R.M., *Biological marker in breast carcinomas: II Clinical correlation with human chorionic gonadotropins.* Cancer 1977; 39: 2391

92 Williams, R.R., McIntire, K.R., Waldmann, T.A. et al., *Tumour-associated antigen levels (CEA, HCG, alpha-feto protein) antedating the diagnosis of cancer in the Framingham study.* J. Natl. Cancer Inst. 1977; 58(6): 1547–1551

93 Donaldson, E.S., van Nagell, J.R. Jr., Pursell, S., Gay, E.C., Meeker, W.R., van Kashmiri, R. and deVoorde, J., *Multiple biochemical markers in patients with gynecologic malignancies.* Cancer 1980; 45: 948–953

94 Rutanen, E.M. and Seppala, M., *The HCG-beta sub-unit radioimmunoassay in nontrophoblastic gynecologic tumours.* Cancer 1978; 41: 692–696

95 Stenman, U.H., Alfthan, H., Ranta, T., Vartiainen, E., Jalkanen, J. and Seppälä, M., *Serum levels of human chorionic gonadotropin in non-pregnant women and men are modulated by gonadotropin-releasing hormone and sex steroids.* J. Clin. Endocrinol. Metab. 1987; 64: 730–736

96 Acevedo, H.F., Cancer 1992; 69: 1818–1828

97 Acevedo, H.F., Cancer 1992; 69: 1829-1842

98 Hernan F. Acevedo, Jennifer Y. Tong., Robert J. Hartsock, *Cancer Human Chorionic Gonadotropin-Beta Sub-unit Gene Expression in Cultured Human Fetal and Cancer Cells of Different Types and Origins.* Cancer 1995; 76: 1467–75

99 Stenman, U.H., Alfthan, H. and Hotakainen, K., *Human chorionic gonadotropin in cancer.* Clin. Biochem. 2004; 37: 549–561

100 Ulf-Håkan Stenman, Aila Tiitinen, Henrik Alfthan, and Leena Valmu, *The classification, functions and clinical use of different isoforms of HCG.* Hum. Reprod. Update 2006; 12(6): 769–784

101 Acevedo, H.F., Krichevsky, A., Campbell-Acevedo, E.A., Galyon, J.C., Buffo, M.J., Hartsock, R.J., *Flow cytometry method for the analysis of membrane-associated human chorionic gonadotropin, its sub-units, and fragments on human cancer cells.* Cancer 1992; 69: 1818–1828

102 Acevedo, H.F, Krichevsky, A., Campbell-Acevedo, E.A., Galyon, J.C., Buffo, M.J., Hartsock, R.J., *Expression of membrane-associated human chorionic gonadotropin, its sub-units, and fragments by cultured human cancer cells.* Cancer 1992; 69: 1829–42

103 Acevedo, H.F., Tong, J.Y., Hartsock, R.J., *Human chorionic gonadotropin-beta sub-unit gene statement in cultured human fetal and cancer cells of different types and angina.* Cancer 1995; 76: 1467–1475

104 Acevedo, H.F. and Robert J. Hartsock, *Metastatic phenotype correlates with high expression of membrane-associated complete β-human chorionic gonadotropin in vivo.* Cancer 1996; 78: 2388–99

105 R.K. Iles, *Ectopic HCG-beta expression by epithelial cancer: Malignant behaviour, metastasis and inhibition of tumour cell apoptosis.* Molecular Cell Endocrin. 2007; 260-262: 264–270

106 *American Cancer Society: Cancer Facts and Figures 2012.* Atlanta, GA, American Cancer Society 2012

[107] L. Kenny, J.J. McAleer, *Elevated serum B-HCG due to a tumour of unknown origin.* Ulster Med. J. 2004; 73(1): 47–49

[108] Toshikazu Uchida, Toshio Shikata, Shin-Ichi Shimizu, Yukie Takimoto, Shiro Iino, Hiroshi Suzuki, Toshitsugu Oda, Kazuyuki Hirano, Mamoru Sugiura, *Gonadotropin and alkaline phosphatase producing occult gastric carcinoma with widespread metastasis of generalized bone.* Cancer 1981; 48(1): 140–150

[109] Acevedo, H.F., Hartsock, R.J., Maroon, J.C., *Detection of membrane-associated human chorionic gonadotropin and its sub-units on human cultured cancer cells of the nervous system.* Cancer Detect. and Prevent. 1997; 21(4): 295–303

[110] Jun Shinoda, Noboru Sakai, Hirohito Yano, Tatsuaki Hattori, Akio Ohkuma and Heima Sakaguchi, *Prognostic Factors and Therapeutic Problems of Primary Intracranial Choriocarcinoma/Germ-Cell Tumours with High Levels of HCG.* J. Neuro-Oncology 2004; 66(1-2): 225–240

[111] Tormey, D.C., Waalkes, T.P., Ahmann, D., Gehrke, C.W., Zumwatt, R.W., Snyder, J. and Hansen, H., *Biological markers in breast carcinoma. I. Incidence of abnormalities of CEA, HCG, three polyamines, and three minor nucleosides.* Cancer 1975; 35: 1095–1100

[112] Dave S.B. Hoon, Terry Sarantou, Fukashi Do, Dorcas D.J. Chi, Christine Kuo, Andrew J. Conrad, Peter Schmid, Roderick Turner, Armando Guiliano, *Detection of metastatic breast cancer by β-HCG polymerase chain reaction.* Int. J. Cancer 1996; 69(5): 369–374

[113] Scholl, P.D., Jurco, S., Austin, J.R., *Ectopic production of beta HCG by a maxillary squamous cell carcinoma.* Head Neck 1997; 19: 701–5

[114] R.A Crawford, R.K. Iles, P.G. Carter, C.J. Caldwell, J.H. Shepherd, T. Chard, *The prognostic significance of beta human chorionic gonadotrophin and its metabolites in women with cervical carcinoma.* J. Clin. Pathol. 1998; 51: 685–688

[115] E.S. Donaldson, J.R. van Nagell Jr., S. Pursell, E.C. Gay, W.R. Meeker, R. Kashmiri, J. van Devoorde, *Multiple biochemical markers in patients with gynecologic malignancies.* Cancer 1980; 45(5): 948–953

[116] M. Carpelan-Holmström, C. Haglund, J. Lundin, H. Alfthan, U.H. Stenman, and P.J. Roberts, *Independent prognostic value of preoperative serum markers CA 242, specific tissue polypeptide antigen and human chorionic gonadotrophin beta, but not of carcinoembryonic antigen or tissue polypeptide antigen in colorectal cancer.* Br. J. Cancer 1996; 74(6): 925–929

[117] T. Shah, R. Srirajaskanthan, M. Bhogal, C. Toubanakis, T. Meyer, A. Noonan, C. Witney-Smith, T. Amin, P. Bhogal, N. Sivathasan, B. Warner, D. Hochhauser, M. E. Caplin, *α-Fetoprotein and human chorionic gonadotrophin-β as prognostic markers in neuroendocrine tumour patients.* Brit. J. Cancer 2008; 99: 72–77

118 Alfthan, H., Haglund, C., Roberts, P., Stenman, U.H., *Elevation of free beta sub-unit of human choriogonadotropin and core beta fragment of human choriogonadotropin in the serum and urine of patients with malignant pancreatic and biliary disease.* Cancer Res. 1992; 52(17): 4628–33

119 Braunstein, G.D., Kamdar, V.V., Kanabus, J. and Rasor, J., *Properties of human chorionic gonadotropin produced in vitro by ovarian carcinoma cells.* J. Clin. Endocrinol. Metab. 1978; 47: 326–332

120 Donaldson, E.S., van Nagell, J.R. Jr., Pursell, S., Gay, E.C., Meeker, W.R., van Kashmiri, R. and deVoorde, J., *Multiple biochemical markers in patients with gynaecological malignancies.* Cancer 1980; 45: 948–953

121 Cauchi, M.N., Koh, S.H., Lim, D. and Hay, D.L., *Oncofoetal antigens in cancer of the cervix and ovary.* Br. J. Cancer 1981; 44: 403–409

122 Grossmann, M., Hoermann, R., Gocze, P.M., Ott, M., Berger, P. and Mann, K., *Measurement of human chorionic gonadotropin-related immunoreactivity in serum, ascites and tumour cysts of patients with gynaecologic malignancies.* Eur. J. Clin. Invest. 1995; 25: 867–873

123 Nozawa, S., Engvall, E., Kano, S., Kurihara, S. and Fishman, W.H., *Sodium butyrate produces concordant expression of 'early placental' alkaline phosphatase, pregnancy-specific beta 1-glycoprotein and human chronic gonadotropin beta-sub-unit in a newly established uterine cervical cancer cell line (SKG-IIIa).* Int. J. Cancer 1983; 32: 267–272

124 Hussa, R.O., Fein, H.G., Pattillo, R.A., Nagelberg, S.B., Rosen, S.W., Weintraub, B.D., Perini, F., Ruddon, R.W. and Cole, L.A., *A distinctive form of human chorionic gonadotropin beta-sub-unit-like material produced by cervical carcinoma cells.* Cancer Res. 1986; 46: 1948–1954

125 Papapetrou, P.D. and Nicopoulou, S.C., *The origin of a human chorionic gonadotropin beta-sub-unit-core fragment excreted in the urine of patients with cancer.* Acta Endocrinol (Copenh.) 1986; 112: 415–422

126 Cole, L.A., Wang, Y.X., Elliott, M., Latif, M., Chambers, J.T., Chambers, S.K. and Schwartz, P.E., *Urinary human chorionic gonadotropin free beta-sub-unit and beta-core fragment: a new marker of gynecological cancers.* Cancer Res. 1988; 48: 1356–1360

127 Norman, R.J., Buck, R.H., Aktar, B., Mayet, N. and Moodley, J., *Detection of a small molecular species of human chorionic gonadotropin in the urine of patients with carcinoma of the cervix and cervical intraepithelial neoplasia: comparison with other assays for human chorionic gonadotropin and its fragments.* Gynecol. Oncol. 1990; 37: 254–259

128 Norman, R.J., de Medeiros, S., Amato, F., Davis, G. and Davy, M., *Beta-core fragment of human chorionic gonadotropin in cervical intraepithelial neoplasia (CIN).* Gynecol. Oncol. 1993; 49: 16–18

[129] Carter, P.G., Iles, R.K., Neven, P., Ind, T.E., Shepherd, J.H. and Chard, T., *The prognostic significance of urinary beta core fragment in premenopausal women with carcinoma of the cervix.* Gynecol. Oncol. 1994: 55: 271–276

[130] Crawford, R.A., Iles, R.K., Carter, P.G., Caldwell, C.J., Shepherd, J.H. and Chard, T., *The prognostic significance of beta human chorionic gonadotrophin and its metabolites in women with cervical carcinoma.* J. Clin. Pathol. 1998; 51: 685–688

[131] Carter, P.G., Iles, R.K., Neven, P., Ind, T.E., Shepherd, J.H. and Chard, T., *Measurement of urinary beta core fragment of human chorionic gonadotrophin in women with vulvovaginal malignancy and its prognostic significance.* Br. J. Cancer 1995; 71: 350–353

[132] Vartiainen, J., Lehtovirta, P., Finne, P., Stenman, U.H. and Alfthan, H., *Preoperative serum concentration of HCGbeta as a prognostic factor in ovarian cancer.* Int. J. Cancer 2001; 95: 313–316

[133] E.S. Donaldson, J.R. van Nagell Jr., S. Pursell, E.C. Gay, W.R. Meeker, R. Kashmiri, J. van Devoorde, *Multiple biochemical markers in patients with gynecologic malignancies.* Cancer 1980; 45(5): 948–953

[134] Justin H. Turner, Hillary Ross, Jeremy Richmon, *Secretion of β-HCG from squamous cell carcinomas of the head and neck.* Otolaryngology Head Neck Surg. 2010; 143: 169–170

[135] Acevedo, H.F., Hartsock, R.J., Maroon, J.C., *Detection of membrane-associated human chorionic gonadotropin and its sub-units on human cultured cancer cells of the nervous system.* Cancer Detect. and Prevent. 1997; 21(4): 295–303

[136] Fraternali-Orcioni, G., Falini, B., Quaini, F., Campo, E., Piccioli, M., Gamberi, B., Pasquinelli, G., Poggi, S., Ascani, S., Sabattini, E., Pileri, S.A., *Beta-HCG aberrant expression in primary mediastinal large B-cell lymphoma.* Am. J. Surg. Pathol. 1999; 23(6): 717–21

[137] Leong, M.Y., English, M., McMullan, D., Ramani, P., *Aberrant expression of beta-HCG in anaplastic large cell lymphoma.* Pediatr. Dev. Pathol. 2008; 11(3): 230–4

[138] Yasuni Nakanuma, Masashi Unoura, Hiroshi Noto, Goroku Ohta, *Human chorionic gonadotropin in primary liver carcinoma in adults.* Virchows Archiv A 1986; 40(3): 365–373

[139] Beach, R., Betts, P., Radford, M., Millward-Sadler, H., *Production of human chorionic gonadotropin by a hepablastoma resulting in precocious puberty.* J. Clin. Path. 1984; 37: 734–737

[140] Braunstein, G.D., Vogel, C.L., Vaitukaitis, J.L., Ross, G.T., *Ectopic production of HCG in Ugandan patients with hepatocellular carcinoma.* Cancer 1973; 32: 223–226

141 Junji Yoshida, Kanji Nagai, Mitsuyo Nishimura, Kenro Takahashi, Ryutaro Kakinuma, Yutaka Nishiwaki, Tomoyuki Yokose, *Secretion of HCG/β-HCG by Squamous Cell Carcinoma of the Lung in a 31-year-old Female Smoker.* Jpn. J. Clin. Oncol. 2000; 30 (3):163–166

142 P. Sagaster, N. Zojer, G. Dekan, H. Ludwig, *A paraneoplastic syndrome mimicking extrauterine pregnancy.* Ann. Oncol. 2002; 13 (1): 170–172

143 Stephan Dirnhofer, Martin Freund, Hermann Rogatsch, Simone Krabichler, Peter Berger, *Selective expression of trophoblastic hormones by lung carcinoma: Neuroendocrine tumours exclusively produce human chorionic gonadotropin [alpha]-sub-unit (HCG[alpha]).* Human Pathology 2000; 31(8): 966–972

144 Saakshi Khattri, Abhirami Vivekanandarajah, Seema Varma, Frank Kong, *Secretion of beta-human chorionic gonadotropin by non-small cell lung cancer: a case report.* J. Med. Case Reports 2011; 5: 19

145 M. Szturmowicz, J. Slodkowska, J. Zych, P. Rudzinski, A. Sakowicz, E. Rowinska-Zakrzewska, *Frequency and Clinical Significance of β-Sub-unit Human Chorionic Gonadotropin Expression in Non-Small Cell Lung Cancer Patients.* Tumour Biol. 1999; 20(2): 99–104

146 Doi, F., Chi, D.D., Charuworn, B.B., Conrad, A.J., Russell, J., Morton, D.L., Hoon, D.S., *Detection of beta-human chorionic gonadotropin mRNA as a marker for cutaneous malignant melanoma.* Int. J. Cancer 1996; 65(4): 454–9

147 Burdick, C.O., *HCG positive mesothelioma.* Am. J. Surg. Pathol. 1993; 17(7): 749–50

148 Okamoto, H., Matsuno, Y., Noguchi, M., Morinaga, S., Fujioka, Y., Tsuchiya, R., Tamura, T., Shimosato, Y., *Malignant pleural mesothelioma producing human chorionic gonadotropin. Report of two cases.* Am. J. Surg. Pathol. 1992; 16(10): 969–74

149 Rich, S., Presant, C.A., Meyer, J., Stevens, S.C., Carr, D., *Human chorionic gonadotropin and malignant mesothelioma.* Cancer 1979; 43(4): 1457–62

150 Stephen P. Slone, Zakaria Ahmed, Laurence A. Cole, Ronald J. Elin, Alvin W. Martin, Roger H. Herzig, Geoffrey P. Herzig, James J. Miller, *Positive Pregnancy Tests in a Nongravid, Premenopausal Woman Due to HCG-Chain Production by Multiple Myeloma.* Am. J. Clin. Pathol. 2005; 124: 108–112

151 Tageja, N., Valent, J., Giorgadze, T., Bentley, G., Zonder, J., *Positive pregnancy tests in a postmenopausal woman due to beta-human chorionic gonadotropin production by multiple myeloma.* Am. J. Med. Sci. 2010; 339(2): 182–4

[152] Hideki Kuroda, Masaki Mandai, Ikuo Konishi, Yasuichiro Yura, Yuko Tsuruta, Atia A. Hamid, Kanako Nanbu, Katsuko Matsushita, Takahide Mori, *Human chorionic gonadotropin (HCG) inhibits cisplatin-induced apoptosis in ovarian cancer cells: Possible role of up-regulation of insulin-like growth factor-1 by HCG.* Int. J. Cancer; 76(4): 571–578

[153] M.R. Rubin, J.P. Bilezikian, S. Birken, Steven Birken and Shonni H. Silverberg, *Human chorionic gonadotropin measurements in parathyroid carcinoma.* J. Endocrinology 1994; 134: 1139–1145

[154] Kahn, C.R., Rosen, S.W., Weintraub, B.D., Fajans, S.S., Gorden, P., *Ectopic production of chorionic gonadotropin and its sub-units by islet-cell tumours.* N. Engl. J. Med. 1977; 297: 565–569

[155] K.N. Syrigos, I. Fyssas, M.M. Konstandoulakis, K.J. Harrington, S. Papadopoulos, N. Milingos, P. Peveretos, B.C. Golematis, *Beta human chorionic gonadotropin concentrations in serum of patients with pancreatic adenocarcinoma.* Gut 1998; 42: 88–91

[156] Philipp U. Heitz, Marlis Kasper, Gunter Kloppel, Julia M. Polak, Judith L. Vaitukaitis, *Glycoprotein-hormone alpha-chain production by pancreatic endocrine tumours: A specific marker for malignancy. Immunocytochemical analysis of tumours of 155 patients.* Cancer 1983; 51(2): 277–282

[157] Henrik Alfthan, Caj Haglund, Peter Roberts, Ulf-Håkan Stenman, *Elevation of Free β Sub-unit of Human Choriogonadotropin and Core β Fragment of Human Choriogonadotropin in the Serum and Urine of Patients with Malignant Pancreatic and Biliary Disease.* Cancer Res. 1992; 52: 4628

[158] Philipp U. Heitz, Marlis Kasper, Gunter Kloppel, Julia M. Polak, Judith L. Vaitukaitis, *Glycoprotein-hormone alpha-chain production by pancreatic endocrine tumours: A specific marker for malignancy. Immunocytochemical analysis of tumours of 155 patients.* Cancer 1983; 51(2): 277–282

[159] Louhimo, J., Alfthan, H., Stenman, U-H., Haglund, C., *Serum HCGβ and CA 72-4 are Stronger Prognostic Factors than CEA, CA 19-9 and CA 242 in Pancreatic Cancer.* Oncology 2004; 66: 126–131

[160] C. Ronald Kahn, MD, Saul W. Rosen, MD, Bruce D. Weintraub, MD, Stefan S. Fajans, MD and Phillip Gorden, MD, *Ectopic Production of Chorionic Gonadotropin and Its Sub-units by Islet-Cell Tumours–A Specific Marker for Malignancy.* N. Engl. J. Med. 1977; 297: 565–569

[161] M.T. Sheaff, J.E. Martin, D.F. Badenoch, S.I. Baithun, *Beta HCG as a prognostic marker in adenocarcinoma of the prostate.* J. Clin. Pathol. 1996; 49(4): 329–332

[162] Eiichi Tahara, Hisao Ito, Kazuhiko Nakagami, Fumio Shimamoto, Masami Yamamoto MD, Kozo Sumii, *Scirrhous argyrophil cell carcinoma of the stomach with multiple production of polypeptide hormones, amine, CEA, lysozyme, and HCG.* Cancer 1982; 49(9): 1904–1915

163 Toshikazu Uchida, Toshio Shikata, Shin-Ichi Shimizu, Yukie Takimoto, Shiro Iino, Hiroshi Suzuki, Toshitsugu Oda, Kazuyuki Hirano, Mamoru Sugiura, *Gonadotropin and alkaline phosphatase producing occult gastric carcinoma with widespread metastasis of generalized bone.* Cancer 1981; 48(1): 140–150

164 Sakaguchi, N., Yoshimura, M., Hershman, J.M., Nishikawa, M., Inada, M., *Paracrine effect of human chorionic gonadotropin ectopically produced from papillary thyroid cancer cells on growth and function of FRTL-5 rat thyroid cells.* Thyroid 1997; 7(5): 779–82

165 Gillott, D.J., Iles, R.K. and Chard, T., *The effects of beta-human chorionic gonadotrophin on the in vitro growth of bladder cancer cell lines.* Br. J. Cancer 1996; 73: 323–326

166 Butler, S.A., Staite, E.M. and Iles, R.K., *Reduction of bladder cancer cell growth in response to HCGbeta CTP37 vaccinated mouse serum.* Oncol. Res. 2003; 14:93–100

167 Pectasides, D., Bafaloucos, D., Antoniou, F., Gogou, L., Economides, N., Varthalitis, J., Dimitriades, M., Kosmidis, P., Athanassiou, A., *TPA, TATI, CEA, AFP, [beta]-HCG, PSA, SCC, and CA 19-9 for Monitoring Transitional Cell Carcinoma of the Bladder.* Amer. J. Clin. Oncology 1996; 19(3): 271–277

168 D.J. Gillott, R.K. Iles and T. Chard. *The effects of beta-human chorionic gonadotrophin on the in vitro growth of bladder cancer cell lines.* Br. J. Cancer 1996 February; 73(3): 323–326

169 B.J. Jenkins, J.E. Martin, S.I. Baithun, R.J. Zuk, R.T.D. Oliver, J.P. Blandy, *Prediction of Response to Radiotherapy in Invasive Bladder Cancer.* British J. Urology 1990; 65(4): 345–348

170 G. Moutzouris, D. Yannopoulos, C. Barbatis, A. Zaharof, Ch. Theodorou, *Is beta-Human Chorionic Gonadotrophin Production by Transitional Cell Carcinoma of the Bladder a Marker of Aggressive Disease and Resistance to Radiotherapy?* British Journal of Urology 1993; 72(6): 907–909

171 Oliver, R.T., Stephenson, C., Collino, C.E., Parkinson, M.C., *Clinicopathological significance of immunoreactive beta-HCG production by bladder cancer.* Mol. Biother. 1988; 1(1): 43–5

172 Z.F. Dobrowolski, B Byrska, M Dolezal, *Prognostic Value of Beta Human Chorionic Gonadotrophin in Blood Serum of Patients with Urinary Bladder Tumours.* Int. J. Urol. Nephrol. 1994; 26(3): 301–306

173 Mohammed Iyoob, Mohammed Ilyas, Gareth D.H. Turner and David Cranston, *Human chorionic gonadotropin-secreting clear cell renal cell carcinoma with paraneoplastic gynaecomastia.* Scand. J. Urol. and Nephrol. 2008; 42(6): 555–557

174 Burçin Tuna, Kutsal Yörükoğlu, Uğur Mungan and Ziya Kirkali, *Urothelial carcinoma of the bladder with trophoblastic differentiation: A case report.* Int. J. Urol. and Nephrol. 2004; 36(4): 529–531

[175] Cole, L.A., Kardana, A., Ying, F.C. and Birken, S., *The biological and clinical significance of nicks in human chorionic gonadotropin and its free beta-sub-unit.* Yale J. Biol. Med. 1991; 6: 627–637

[176] Cole, L.A., Birken, S., Sutphen, S., Hussa, R.O. and Pattillo, R.A., *Absence of the COOH-terminal peptide on ectopic human chorionic gonadotropin beta-sub-unit (HCG beta).* Endocrinology 1982; 110: 2198–2200

[177] Ascheim, S. and Zondek, B., *Das Hormon des Hypophysenvorderlappens: testobjekt zum nachweis des hormons.* Klin. Wochenschr. 1927; 6: 248–252

[178] Wide, L. and Gemzell, C.A., *An immunological pregnancy test.* Acta Endocrinol (Copenh.) 1960; 35: 261–267

[179] Vaitukaitis, J.L., Braunstein, G.D. and Ross, G.T., *A radioimmunoassay which specifically measures human chorionic gonadotropin in the presence of human luteinizing hormone.* Am. J. Obstet. Gynecol. 1972; 113: 751–758

[180] Stenman, U-H., Alfthan, H. and Hotakainen, K., *Human chorionic gonadotropin in cancer.* Clin. Biochem. 2004; 37: 549–561

[181] Stenman, U-H., Bidart, J.M., Birken, S., Mann, K., Nisula, B. and O'Connor, J., *Standardization of protein immunoprocedures. Choriogonadotropin (CG).* Scand. J. Clin. Lab. Invest. Suppl. 1993; 216: 42–78

[182] Ulf-Håkan Stenman, Aila Tiitinen, Henrik Alfthan and Leena Valmu, *The classification, functions and clinical use of different isoforms of HCG.* Hum. Reprod. Update 2006; 12(6): 769–784

[183] Navarro, M., *72nd Science Meeting of the Cavite Med. Soc.* 1959; Trece Martires City, Philippines

[184] Richard A. McPherson, Matthew R. Pincus, *Henry's Clinical Diagnosis and Management by Laboratory Methods (21st ed.)* 2006; Philadelphia, Saunders. ISBN: 1-4160-0287-1

[185] www.caprofile.net

[186] Emil K. Schandl, *The Cancer Profile and its Clinical Application.* Townsend Letter, 2010, Aug/Sept

[187] Contractor, S.F., Davies, H., *Effect of human chorionic somatomammotrophin on phytohaemagglutin-induced lymphocyte transformation.* Nature 1973; 243: 284

[188] Kayisli, U., Selam, B., Guzeloglu-Kayisli, O., Demir, R., Arici, A., *Human chorionic gonadotropin contributes to maternal immunotolerance and endometrial apoptosis by regulating Fas-Fas ligand system.* J. Immunol. 2003; 171(5): 2305–13

[189] McManus, L.M., Naughton, N.A., Martinex, H.A.A., *Human chorionic gonadotropin in human neoplastic cells.* Cancer Res. 1976; 36: 3476

[190] G. Moutzouris, D. Yannopoulos, C. Barbatis, A. Zaharof, Ch. Theodorou, *Is beta-Human Chorionic Gonadotrophin Production by Transitional Cell Carcinoma of the Bladder a Marker of Aggressive Disease and Resistance to Radiotherapy?* British J. Urology 1993; 72(6): 907–909

[191] Stenman, U-H., Alfthan, H. and Hotakainen, K., *Human chorionic gonadotropin in cancer.* Clin. Biochem. 2004; 37: 549–561

[192] B.J. Jenkins, J.E. Martin, S.I. Baithun, R.J. Zuk, R.T.D. Oliver, J.P. Blandy, *Prediction of Response to Radiotherapy in Invasive Bladder Cancer.* British J. Urology 1990; 65(4): 345–348

[193] Oliver, R.T., Stephenson, C., Collino, C.E., Parkinson, M.C., *Clinicopathological significance of immunoreactive beta-HCG production by bladder cancer.* Mol. Biother. 1988; 1(1): 43–5

[194] R.K. Iles, B.J. Jenkins, R.T.D. Oliver, J.P. Blandy, T. Chard, *Beta Human Chorionic Gonadotrophin in Serum and Urine. A Marker for Metastatic Urothelial Cancer.* B. J. Urol. 1989; 63(3): 241–244

[195] J.E. Martin, B.J. Jenkins, R.J. Zuk, R.T.D. Oliver and S.I. Baithun, *Human chorionic gonadotrophin expression and histological findings as predictors of response to radiotherapy in carcinoma of the bladder.* Virchows Archiv. 1989; 414(3): 273–277

[196] Schandl, E.K., *The cancer profile and its clinical applications.* Townsend Newsletter 2010; Aug-Sept

[197] Zygmunt, M., Herr, F., Keller-Schoenwetter, S., Kunzi-Rapp, K., Münstedt, K., Rao, C.V., Lang, U., Preissner. K.T., *Characterization of human chorionic gonadotropin as a novel angiogenic factor.* J. Clin. Endocrinol. Metab. 2002; 87(11): 5290–6

[198] Hideki Kuroda, Masaki Mandai, Ikuo Konishi, Yasuichiro Yura, Yuko Tsuruta, Atia A. Hamid, Kanako Nanbu, Katsuko Matsushita, Takahide Mori, *Human chorionic gonadotropin (HCG) inhibits cisplatin-induced apoptosis in ovarian cancer cells: Possible role of up-regulation of insulin-like growth factor-1 by HCG.* Int. J. Cancer; 76(4): 571–578

[199] K.N. Syrigos, I. Fyssas, M.M. Konstandoulakis, K.J. Harrington, S. Papadopoulos, N. Milingos, P. Peveretos, B.C. Golematis, *Beta human chorionic gonadotropin concentrations in serum of patients with pancreatic adenocarcinoma.* Gut 1998; 42: 88–91

[200] Regelson, W., *Have we found the 'definitive cancer biomarker'? The diagnostic and therapeutic implications of human chorionic gonadotropin-beta statement as a key to malignancy.* Cancer 1995; 76: 1299–1301

[201] Srivastava, P., Russo, J. and Russo, I.H., *Chorionic gonadotropin inhibits rat mammary carcinogenesis through activation of programmed cell death.* Carcinogenesis 1997; 18: 1799–180

[202] Hamada, A.L., Nakabayashi, K., Sato, A., Kiyoshi, K., Takamatsu, Y., Laoag-Fernandez, J.B., O'Hara, N. and Maruo, T., *Transfection of antisense chorionic gonadotropin beta gene into choriocarcinoma cells suppresses the cell proliferation and induces apoptosis.* J. Clin. Endocrinol. Metab. 2005; 90: 4873–4879

[203] Butler, S.A. and Iles, R.K., *The free monomeric beta sub-unit of human chorionic gonadotrophin (HCG beta) and the recently identified homodimeric beta-beta sub-unit (HCG beta beta) both have autocrine growth effects.* Tumour Biol. 2004; 25: 18–23

[204] Acavedo, H.F. et al., *Flow cytometry method for the analysis of membrane-associated HCG, its sub-units and fragments on human cancer cells.* Cancer 1992; 69: 1818–1828

[205] Acavedo, H.F. et al., *HCG-β gene expression in cultured human fetal and cancer cells.* Cancer 1995; 76: 1467–1475

[206] Marcillac, I. et al., *Free human chorionic gonadotropin β sub-unit in gonadal and non-gonadal neoplasms.* Cancer Res. 1992; 52: 3901–3907

[207] Martinez Flores, A. et al., *Development and validation of an in vitro culture model for the study of the differentiation of human trophoblast.* [In Spanish.] Ginecol. Obstet. Mex. 2006; 74(12): 657–665

[208] Bjurlin, M.A. et al., *Histological pure seminoma with an elevated beta-HCG of 4497IU/l.* Urology 2007; 70(5): 1007

[209] Warburg, O., *On the origin of cancer cells.* Science 1956; 123(3191): 309–14

[210] Warburg, O., *On the origin of cancer cells.* Science 1956; 123(3191): 309–14

[211] Otto Warburg, *The Prime Cause and Prevention of Cancer.* Lecture to Nobel Laureates, 1966, June 30

[212] http://healingtools.tripod.com/primecause1.html

[213] José M. Cuezva, Maryla Krajewska, Miguel López de Heredia, Stanislaw Krajewski, Gema Santamaría, Hoguen Kim, Juan M. Zapata, Hiroyuki Marusawa, Margarita Chamorro and John C. Reed, *The bioenergetic signature of cancer, a marker of tumour progression.* Cancer Research 2002; 62: 6674–6681

[214] John, A.P., *Dysfunctional mitochondria, not oxygen insufficiency, cause cancer cells to produce inordinate amounts of lactic acid: the impact of this on the treatment of cancer.* Med. Hypothesis 2001; 57(4): 429–432

[215] Muniswamy Madesh, Lakshmi Bhaskar and K.A. Balasubramanian, *Enterocyte viability and mitochondrial function after graded intestinal ischemia and reperfusion in rats.* Moll. and Cell Biochem. 1997; 167(1-2): 81–87

[216] Robert A. Gatenby and Robert J. Gillies, *Why do cancers have high aerobic glycolysis?* Nature Reviews Cancer 2004; 4: 891–899

[217] Seyfried, T.N., Shelton, L.M., *Cancer as a metabolic disease.* Nutr. Metab. (Lond.) 2010; 27-7: 7

[218] Rucker, R.R. and Mueller, G.C., *Effect of Oxygen Tension on HeLa Cell Growth.* Cancer Res. 1960; 20: 944

[219] Lohmann, K., Biochem. Z., 1933: 262

[220] Dobashi, Y., Watanabe, H., *Differential expression and pathological significance of autocrine motility factor/glucose-6-phosphate isomerase expression in human lung carcinomas.* J. Pathol. 2006; 210 (4): 431–40

[221] Watanabe, H, Takehana, K, Date, M., Shinozaki, T., Raz, A., *Tumour cell autocrine motility factor is the neuroleuk.in/phosphohexose isomerase polypeptide.* Cancer Res. 1996; 56 (13): 2960–3

[222] Lance A. Liottaab, Raya Mandlerc, Genesio Muranoc, *Tumour cell autocrine motility factor.* Proc. Natl. Acad. Sci. USA 1986; 83: 3302–3306

[223] Hideomi Watanabe, Kenji Takehana, Masayo Date, Tetsuya Shinozaki, Avraham Raz, *Tumour Cell Autocrine Motility Factor Is the Neuroleukin/Phosphohexose Isomerase Polypeptide.* Cancer Res. 1996; 56: 2960

[224] T. Yanagawa, T. Funasaka, S. Tsutsumi, H. Watanabe and A. Raz, *Novel roles of the autocrine motility factor/phosphoglucose isomerase in tumour malignancy.* Endocrine Related Cancer 2005; 11 (4): 749–759

[225] Shengyun Fang, Marco Ferrone, Cuihong Yang, Jane P. Jensen, Swati Tiwari, Allan M. Weissman, *The tumour autocrine motility factor receptor, gp78, is a ubiquitin protein ligase implicated in degradation from the endoplasmic reticulum.* Lab. Invest. 2004; 84(4): 513–22

[226] Yanagawa, T., Watanabe, H., Takeuchi, T., Fujimoto, S., Kurihara, H., Takagishi, K., *Overexpression of autocrine motility factor in metastatic tumour cells: possible association with augmented expression of KIF3A and GDI-beta.* Lab. Invest. 2004; 84(4): 513–22

[227] Haga, A., Funasaka, T., Niinaka, Y., Raz, A., Nagase, H., *Autocrine motility factor signaling induces tumour apoptotic resistance by regulations Apaf-1 and Caspase-9 apoptosome expression.* Int. J. Cancer 2003; 107(5): 707–14

[228] T. Yanagawa, T. Funasaka, S. Tsutsumi, H. Watanabe, A. Raz, *Novel roles of the autocrine motility factor/phosphoglucose isomerase in tumour malignancy.* Endocr. Relat. Cancer 2004; (11): 749–759

[229] Funasaka, T., Raz, A., *The role of autocrine motility factor in tumour and tumour microenvironment.* Cancer Metastasis Rev. 2007; 26(3-4): 725–35

[230] Baumann, M., Kappl, A., Lang, T., Brand, K., Siegfried, W., Paterok, E., *The diagnostic validity of the serum tumour marker phosphohexose isomerase (PHI) in patients with gastrointestinal, kidney, and breast cancer.* Cancer Invest. 1990; 8(3-4): 351–6

231 Hecht, F.M., Busch, M.P., Rawal, B., Webb, M., Rosenberg, E., Swanson, M., Chesney, M., Anderson, J., Levy, J., Kahn, J.O., *Use of laboratory tests and clinical symptoms for identification of primary HIV infection.* AIDS 2002; 16(8): 1119–29

232 Bodansky, O., *Serum Phosphohexose isomerase in cancer. I. Method of determination and establishment of range of normal values.* Cancer 1954; 7: 1191

233 Damle, S.R., Talavdekar, R.V., Panse, T.B., *The studies on glycolytic enzymes in relation to cancer. II. Comparative study of phosphohexose-isomerase, aldolase, isocitric dehydrogenase, serum glutamic oxaloacetic and pyruvic transaminase, and alkaline phosphatase in liver.* Indian J. Cancer 1971; 8(1): 21–9

234 Anokhin, V.N., *Use of coefficients of enzymatic activity for differential diagnosis of liver diseases.* Lab. Delo. 1976; 7: 401–4

235 Harish Goel, G.S. Kohli and Harbans Lal, *Serum phosphohexose isomerase levels in patients with head and neck cancer.* The Journal of Laryngology & Otology 1986; 100: 581–586

236 P.C. Verma, T. Ojha, D. Yadav and D.D. Hemani, *Study of serum phosphohexose isomerase (PHI) levels in the management of head and neck malignancies.* Indian Journal of Otolaryngology and Head & Neck Surgery 2001; 53(1): 40–46

237 Muir, Grainger G., *Possible use of phosphohexose isomerase as a preliminary to exfoliative cytology in screening for cervical carcinoma.* J. Clin. Pathol. 1966; 19(4): 378–383

238 Maity, C., Boo-Chai, Khoo, *Tissue and serum levels of phospho-hexo-isomerase and lactate dehydrogenase in breast cancer patients: Their diagnostic importance.* Plastic & Reconstructive Surgery 1990; 86(3): 614

239 Matthias Baumann, Karl Brand· Josef Giedl, Paul Hermanek, Stefan Ruf, Johannes Scheele, Suse Hoferichter, Franz P. Gall., *Significance of Serum Phosphohexose Isomerase in Gastrointestinal Cancer at Different Stages.* Oncology 1988; 45(3): 153–158

240 M.H. Gault, M.W. Cohen, L.M. Kahana, F.T. Leelin, J.F. Meakins and M. Aronovitch, *Serum enzymes in patients with carcinoma of lung: lactic-acid dehydrogenase, phosphohexose isomerase, alkaline phosphatase and glutamic oxaloacetic transaminase.* Can. Med. Assoc. J. 1967; 96(2): 87–94

241 Grainger G. Muir, *Possible use of phosphohexose isomerase as a preliminary to exfoliative cytology in screening for cervical carcinoma.* J. Clin. Pathol. 1966; 19(4): 378–383

242 Baumann, M, Kappl, A., Lang, T., Brand, K., Siegfried, W., Paterok, E., *The diagnostic validity of the serum tumour marker phosphohexose isomerase (PHI) in patients with gastrointestinal, kidney, and breast cancer.* Cancer Invest. 1990; 8(3-4): 351–6

243 Harish Goel, G.S. Kohli, Harbans Lal, *Serum phosphohexose isomerase levels in patients with head and neck cancer.* J. Laryngology & Otology 1986; 100: 581–586

244 Schandl, E.K., *Clinical laboratory results data bank.* Unpublished, in preparation

245 Hideomi Watanabe, Kenji Takehana, Masayo Date, Tetsuya Shinozaki and Avraham Raz, *Tumour Cell Autocrine Motility Factor Is the Neuroleukin/Phosphohexose Isomerase Polypeptide.* Cancer Res. 1996; 56: 2960

246 T. Yanagawa, T. Funasaka, S. Tsutsumi, H. Watanabe, A. Raz, *Novel roles of the autocrine motility factor/phosphoglucose isomerase in tumour malignancy.* Endocrine-Related Cancer 2004; 11: 749–759

247 T. Yanagawa, T. Funasaka, S. Tsutsumi, H. Watanabe and A. Raz, *Novel roles of the autocrine motility factor/phosphoglucose isomerase in tumour malignancy.* Endocrine-Related Cancer 2004; 11(4): 749–759

248 Haga, A., Funasaka, T., Niinaka, Y., Raz, A, and Nagase, H., *Autocrine motility factor signaling induces tumour apoptotic resistance by regulations Apaf-1 and Caspase-9 apoptosome expression.* Int. J. Cancer 2003; 107: 707–714

249 Folkman, J. and Klagsbrun, M., *Angiogenic factors.* Science 1987; 235: 442–447

250 Folkman, J., *What is the evidence that tumours are angiogenesis dependent?* J. Nat. Cancer Inst. 1990; 82: 4–6

251 Folkman, J. and Shing, Y., *Angiogenesis.* J. Biol. Chem. 1992; 267: 10931–10934

252 Leung, D.W., Cachianes, G., Kuang, W.J., Goeddel, D.V. and Ferrara, N., *Vascular endothelial growth factor is a secreted angiogenic mitogen.* Science 1989; 246: 1306–1309

253 H.M. Pinedo, Dennis J. Slamon, *Translational Research: The Role of VEGF in Tumour Angiogenesis.* The Oncologist 2000; 5(1): 1–2

254 T. Yanagawa, T. Funasaka, S. Tsutsumi, H. Watanabe, A. Raz, *Novel roles of the autocrine motility factor/phosphoglucose isomerase in tumour malignancy.* Endocrine-Related Cancer; 11 (4): 749–759

255 Funasaka, T., Haga, A., Raz, A., Nagase, H., *Tumour autocrine motility factor induces hyperpermeability of endothelial and mesothelial cells leading to accumulation of ascites fluid.* Biochem. Biophys. Res. Commun. 2002; 26; 293(1): 192–200

[256] E.K. Schandl, *The Cancer Profile and its Clinical Application.* Townsend Letter, 2010; Aug/Sept :84–86

[257] R.A.S. Hemat, *Orthomolecularism in Principle and Practice.* Authorhouse, 2004

[258] Landt, S., Jeschke, S., Koeninger, A., Thomas, A., Heusner, T., Korlach, S., Ulm, K., Schmidt, P., Blohmer, J.U., Lichtenegger, W., Sehouli, J., Kuemmel, S., *Tumour-specific correlation of tumour M2 pyruvate kinase in pre-invasive, invasive and recurrent cervical cancer.* Anticancer Res. 2010; 30(2): 375–81

[259] Aslı Hapa, Gül Erkin, Gülşen Hasçelik, Dilara Pektaş, Umut Arslan, *Plasma TM2-PK levels in mycosis fungoides patients.* Archives of Dermatological Research 2011; 303(1): 35–40

[260] Joachim Schneider, Harald Morr, Hans-Georg Velcovsky, Günter Weisse and Erich Eigenbrodt, *Quantitative Detection of Tumour M2-Pyruvate Kinase in Plasma of Patients with Lung Cancer in Comparison to Other Lung Diseases.* Cancer Detection and Prevention 2000; 24(6): 531–535

[261] X.I.E. Feng, G.A.O. Quangeng, W.U. Guoliang et al., *Measurement and clinical significance of serum tumour type M2-pyruvate kinase in patients with gastric cancer.* Jiangsu Med. J. 2006; 10

[262] Hardt, P.D., Ngoumou, B., Rupp, J., Schnell-Kretschmer, H., Klör, H-U., *Tumour M2-PK: A promising tumour marker in the diagnosis of gastrointestinal cancer.* http://www.augen.med.uni-giessen.de/med3/poster/publ_pdf/050.pdf

[263] Pezzilli, R., Migliori, M., Morselli-Labate, A.M., Campana, D., Ventrucci, M., Tomassetti, P., Corinaldesi, R., *Diagnostic value of tumour M2-pyruvate kinase in neuroendocrine tumours. A comparative study with chromogranin.* Anticancer Res. 2003; 23(3C): 2969–72

[264] Board, M., Humm, S., Newsholme, E.A., *Maximum activities of key enzymes of glycolysis, glutaminolysis, pentose phosphate pathway and tricarboxylic acid cycle in normal, neoplastic and suppressed cells.* Biochem. J. 1990; 265(2): 503–9

[265] John C. Chatham, *Lactate – the forgotten fuel!* J. Physiol. 2002; 542: 333

[266] Dewhirst, M.W., *Concepts of oxygen transport at the microcirculatory level.* Semin. Radiat. Oncol. 1998; 8: 143–150

[267] Dewhirst, M.W. *Mechanisms underlying hypoxia development in tumours.* Adv. Exp. Med. Biol. 2003; 510: 51–56

[268] Pierre Sonveaux, Frédérique Végran, Thies Schroeder, Melanie C. Wergin, Julien Verrax, Zahid N. Rabbani, Christophe J. De Saedeleer, Kelly M. Kennedy, Caroline Diepart, Bénédicte F. Jordan, Michael J. Kelley, Bernard Gallez, Miriam L. Wahl, Olivier Feron, Mark W. Dewhirst, *Targeting lactate-fueled respiration selectively kills hypoxic tumor cells in mice.* J. Clin. Invest. 2008; 118(12): 3930–3942

[269] John, A.P., *Dysfunctional mitochondria, not oxygen insufficiency, cause cancer cells to produce inordinate amounts of lactic acid: the impact of this on the treatment of cancer.* Med. Hypotheses 2001; 57(4): 429–31

[270] Brizel, D.M. et al., *Elevated tumour lactate concentrations predict for an increased risk of metastases in head-and-neck cancer.* Int. J. Radiat. Oncol. Biol. Phys. 2001; 51: 349–353

[271] Walenta, S. et al., *Correlation of high lactate levels in head and neck tumours with incidence of metastasis.* Am. J. Pathol. 1997; 150: 409–415

[272] Walenta, S. et al. *High lactate levels predict likelihood of metastases, tumour recurrence, and restricted patient survival in human cervical cancers.* Cancer Res. 2000; 60: 916–921

[273] Jensen, J.A., Hunt, T.K., Scheuenstuhl, H., Banda, M.J., *Effect of lactate, pyruvate, and pH on secretion of angiogenesis and mitogenesis factors by macrophages.* Lab. Invest. 1986; 54(5): 574–8

[274] Hirschhaeuser, F., Sattler, U.G., Mueller-Klieser, W., *Lactate: a metabolic key player in cancer.* Cancer Res. 2011; 71(22): 6921–5

[275] Konstantopoulos, K., Thomas, S.N., *Cancer cells in transit: the vascular interactions of tumour cells.* Ann. Rev. Biomed. Eng. 2009; 11: 177–202

[276] Thomas, S.N., Tong, Z., Stebe, K.J., Konstantopoulos, K., *Identification, characterization and utilization of tumour cell selectin ligands in the design of colon cancer diagnostics.* Biorheology 2009; 46(3): 207–25

[277] Thomas, S.N., Zhu, F., Schnaar, R.L., Alves, C.S., Konstantopoulos, K., *Carcinoembryonic antigen and CD44 variant isoforms co-operate to mediate colon carcinoma cell adhesion to E- and L-selectin in shear flow.* J. Biol. Chem. 2008; 283(23): 15647–55

[278] Hans J. Hansen, Jack J. Snyder, Edward Miller, J.P. Vandevoorde, O. Neal Miller, L.R. Hines, J.J. Burns, *Carcinoembryonic antigen (CEA) assay: A laboratory adjunct in the diagnosis and management of cancer.* Human Path. 1974; 5(2): 139–147

[279] Ando, S., Kimura, H., Iwai, N., Shima, M., Ando, M., Kuriyama, T., *Optimal combination of seven tumour markers in prediction of advanced stage at first examination of patients with non-small cell lung cancer.* Anticancer Research 2001; 21(4B): 3085–3092

[280] Gold, P., Freedman, S.O., *Demonstration of tumour-specific antigens in human colonic carcinomata by immunological tolerance and absorption techniques.* J. Exp. Med. 1965; 121: 439

[281] Hammarstrom, S., *The carcinoembryonic antigen (CEA) family: structures, suggested functions and expression in normal and malignant tissues.* Semin. Cancer Biol. 1999; 9: 67–81

[282] Chatchawan Singhapol, Deepali Pal, Rafal Czapiewski, Mahendar Porika, Glyn Nelson, Gabriele C. Saretzki, *Mitochondrial Telomerase Protects Cancer Cells from Nuclear DNA Damage and Apoptosis.* Plosone 2013; 8(1): e52989

[283] Kovalenko, O.A., Caron, M.J., Lima, P., Medrano, C., Thomas, A.P., Kimura, M., Bonini, M.G., Herbig, U., Santos, J.H., *A mutant telomerase defective in nuclear-cytoplasmic shuttling fails to immortalize cells and is associated with mitochondrial dysfunction.* Aging Cell 2010; 9(2): 203–19

[284] Blackburn, E.H., *Telomeres and telomerase: their mechanisms of action and the effects of altering their functions.* FEBS Lett. 2005; 579 (4): 859–62

[285] Blackburn, K.A., *Telomerase and Cancer.* Kirk A. Landon – AACR Prize for Basic Cancer Research Lecture American Association for Cancer Research 2005

[286] *Pathologic Basis of Disease 8th ed.* 2010: 282

[287] Downward, J., *Targeting RAS signalling pathways in cancer therapy.* Nat. Rev. Cancer 2003; 3(1): 11–22

[288] Witzany, G., *The Viral Origins of Telomeres and Telomerases and their Important Role in Eukaryogenesis and Genome Maintenance.* Biosemiotics 2008; 1: 191–206

[289] Kovalenko, O.A., Kaplunov, J., Herbig, U., Detoledo, S., Azzam, E.I., Santos, J.H., *Expression of (NES-)hTERT in cancer cells delays cell cycle progression and increases sensitivity to genotoxic stress.* PLoS One. 2010; 5(5): e10812

[290] J.W. Shay, R.R. Reddel, W.E. Wright, *Cancer and Telomeres–An alternative to Telomerase Science.* 2012; 336(6087): 1388–1390

[291] Tsao, J., Zhao, Y., Lukas, J., Yang, X., Shah, A., Press, M., Shibata, D., *Telomerase activity in normal and neoplastic breast.* Clin. Cancer Res. 1997; 3(4): 627–31

[292] Epel, E.S., Lin, J., Dhabhar, F.S., Wolkowitz, O.M., Puterman, E., Karan, L., Blackburn, E.H., *Dynamics of telomerase activity in response to acute psychological stress.* Brain Behav. Immun. 2010; 24(4): 531–9

[293] Ahmed, S., Passos, J.F., Birket, M.J., Beckmann, T., Brings, S., Peters, H., Birch-Machin, M.A., von Zglinicki, T., Saretzki, G., *Telomerase does not counteract telomere shortening but protects mitochondrial function under oxidative stress.* J. Cell. Sci. 2008; 121(Pt7): 1046–53

[294] Smith, G., Stubbins, M.J., Harries, L.W., Wolf, C.R., *Molecular genetics of the human cytochrome P450 monooxygenase superfamily.* Xenobiotica 1999; 28 (12): 1129–65

[295] Wood, R., *The discovery of a universal cancer marker.* Int. J. of Phytotherapy 2012; 1(1): 5–8

[296] P. Biava, *Cancer and the Search for Lost Meaning.* North Atlantic Books, 2009

[297] http://americanmetaboliclaboratories.net/CA_Profile-The_Original.html

[298] P. Biava, *Cancer and the Search for Lost Meaning.* North Atlantic Books, 2009

[299] Preetha Anand, Ajaikumar B. Kunnumakara, Chitra Sundaram, Kuzhuvelil B. Harikumar, Sheeja T. Tharakan, Oiki S. Lai, Bokyung Sung and Bharat B. Aggarwal, *Cancer is a Preventable Disease that Requires Major Lifestyle Changes.* Pharm. Res. 2008; 25(9): 2097–2116

[300] http://indiatoday.digitaltoday.in/index.php?option=com_content&task=view &isseid=48&id=6022&sectionid=30&Itemid=1

[301] Fryda, Dr Waltrout, *Adrenalin deficiency as the cause of cancer formation, 4th Edition.* 1987; Kunst and Alltag, Munich; ISBN: 3-88410-079-3

[302] Williams, X.K., *Cancer Concerns.* 2011; Xtra Health Publications, London; ISBN: 978-0-9568552-2-0

[303] Stenman, U.H., Alfthan, H. and Hotakainen, K., *Human chorionic gonadotropin in cancer.* Clin. Biochem. 2004; 37: 549–561

[304] Rotmensch, S. and Cole, L.A., *False diagnosis and needless therapy of presumed malignant disease in women with false-positive human chorionic gonadotropin concentrations.* Lancet 2000; 355: 712–715

[305] Laurence A. Cole, Kirsi M. Rinne, Shohreh Shahabi, Aziza Omrani, *False-Positive HCG Assay Results Leading to Unnecessary Surgery and Chemotherapy and Needless Occurrences of Diabetes and Coma.* Clinical Chemistry 1999; 45(2): 313–314

[306] Yoshimoto, Y., Wolfsen, A.R., Odell, W.D., *Human chorionic gonadotropin-like substance in nonendocrine tissues of normal subjects.* Science 1977; 197(4303): 575–577

[307] Braunstein, G.D., *False-positive serum human chorionic gonadotropin results: causes, characteristics, and recognition.* Am. J. Obstet. Gynecol. 2002; 187: 217–224

[308] Tietz, N.W., *Clinical Guide to Laboratory Tests. Second Edition.* Saunders, 1990

[309] Kricka, L.J., *Human Anti-Animal Antibody Interferences in Immunological Assays.* Clinical Chemistry 1999; 45(7): 942–956

[310] Alfthan, H., Haglund, C., Roberts, P. and Stenman, U-H., *Elevation of free β-sub-unit of human choriogonadotropin and core β fragment of human choriogonadotropin in the serum and urine of patients with malignant pancreatic and biliary disease.* Cancer Res. 1992; 52: 4628–4633

[311] Cole, L.A., Sutton, J.M., Higgins, T.N. and Cembrowski, G.S., *Between-method variation in human chorionic gonadotropin test results.* Clin. Chem. 2004; 50: 874–882

[312] Laurence A. Cole, Kirsi M. Rinne, Shohreh Shahabi, Aziza Omrani, *False-Positive HCG Assay Results Leading to Unnecessary Surgery and Chemotherapy and Needless Occurrences of Diabetes and Coma.* Clinical Chemistry 1999; 45(2): 313–314

[313] Laurence A. Cole, Kirsi M. Rinne, Shohreh Shahabi, Aziza Omrani, *False-Positive HCG Assay Results Leading to Unnecessary Surgery and Chemotherapy and Needless Occurrences of Diabetes and Coma.* Clinical Chem. 1999; 45(2): 313–314

[314] Laurence A. Cole, *Immunoassay of human chorionic gonadotropin, its free subunits, and metabolites.* Clinical Chemistry December 1997; 43(12): 2233–2243

[315] Basbous, J., Knani, D., Bonneaud, N., Giorgi, D., Brondello, J.M., Rouquier, S., *Induction of ASAP (MAP9) contributes to p53 stabilization in response to DNA damage.* Cell Cycle 2012; 11(12): 2380–90

[316] Sengupta, S., Harris, C.C., *p53: traffic cop at the crossroads of DNA repair and recombination.* Nat. Rev. Mol. Cell. Biol. 2005; 6(1): 44–55

[317] Basbous, J., Knani, D., Bonneaud, N., Giorgi, D., Brondello, J.M., Rouquier, S., *Induction of ASAP (MAP9) contributes to p53 stabilization in response to DNA damage.* Cell Cycle 2012; 11(12): 2380–90

[318] Basbous, J., Knani, D., Bonneaud, N., Giorgi, D., Brondello, J.M., Rouquier, S., *Induction of ASAP (MAP9) contributes to p53 stabilization in response to DNA damage.* Cell Cycle 2012; 11(12): 2380–90

[319] Mahata, B., Sundqvist, A., Xirodimas, D.P., *Recruitment of RPL11 at promoter sites of p53-regulated genes upon nucleolar stress through NEDD8 and in an Mdm2-dependent manner.* Oncogene 2012; 31(25): 3060–71

[320] Lee, J.H., Jin, Y., He, G., Zeng, S.X., Wang, Y.V., Wahl, G.M., Lu, H., *Hypoxia activates tumour suppressor p53 by inducing ATR-Chk1 kinase cascade-mediated phosphorylation and consequent 14-3-3γ inactivation of MDMX protein.* J. Biol. Chem. 2012; 287(25): 20898–903

[321] Hollstein, M., Sidransky, D., Vogelstein, B., Harris, C.C., *p53 mutations in human cancers.* Science 1991; 253(5015): 49–53

[322] Reo Maruyama, Minoru Toyota, Hiromu Suzuki, Yasushi Sasaki, Fumio Aoki, Yasuhisa Shinomura, Kohzoh Imai and Takashi Tokino, *The functional relation of vitamin D receptor and p53 in cancer cells.* Cell, Molecular and Tumour Biology: Oncogenes/Tumour Suppressor Genes
http://aacrmeetingabstracts.org/cgi/content/abstract/2006/3/B133

[323] Zhu, H., Mao, Q., Lin, Y., Yang, K., Xie, L., *RNA interference targeting mutant p53 inhibits growth and induces apoptosis in DU145 human prostate cancer cells.* Med. Oncol. 2011; 28(Suppl. 1): S381–7

[324] Blagosklonny, M.V., *p53: An ubiquitous target of anticancer drugs.* International Journal of Cancer 2002; 98: 161–166

[325] Noll, J.E., Jeffery, J., Al-Ejeh, F., Kumar, R., Khanna, K.K., Callen, D.F., Neilsen, P.M., *Mutant p53 drives multinucleation and invasion through a process that is suppressed by ANKRD11.* Oncogene 2012; 31(23): 2836–48

[326] Attias-Geva, Z., Bentov, I., Kidron, D., Amichay, K., Sarfstein, R., Fishman, A., Bruchim, I., Werner, H., *p53 regulates insulin-like growth factor-I receptor gene expression in uterine serous carcinoma and predicts responsiveness to an insulin-like growth factor-I receptor-directed targeted therapy.* Eur. J. Cancer 2012; 48(10): 1570–80

[327] Royds, J.A., Iacopetta, B., *p53 and disease: when the guardian angel fails.* Cell Death Differ 2006; 13(6): 1017–26

[328] Lane, D.P., *Exploiting the p53 pathway for the diagnosis and therapy of human cancer.* Cold Spring Harb. Symp. Quant. Biol. 2005; 70: 489–97

[329] Lorenzo Romero, J.G., Salinas Sánchez, A.S., Giménez Bachs, J.M., Sánchez Sánchez, F., Escribano Martínez, J., Hernández Millán, I.R., Segura Martín, M., Virseda Rodríguez, J.A., *p53 gene mutations in superficial bladder cancer.* Urol. Int. 2004; 73(3): 212–8

[330] Royds, J.A., Iacopetta, B., *p53 and disease: when the guardian angel fails.* Cell Death Differ. 2006; 13(6): 1017–26

[331] T. Takahashi, M.M. Nau, I. Chiba et al., *p53: a frequent target for genetic abnormalities in lung cancer.* Science 1989; 246(4929): 491–494

[332] S.M. Bodner, J.D. Minna, S.M. Jensen et al., *Expression of mutant p53 proteins in lung cancer correlates with the class of p53 gene mutation.* Oncogene 1992; 7(4): 743–749

[333] http://ghr.nlm.nih.gov/gene/TP53

[334] Poornima U. Hegde, Amy C. Brenski, David D. Caldarelli, James Hutchinson, William R. Panje, Nancy B. Wood, Sue Leurgans, Harvey D. Preisler, Samuel G. Taylor, Leslie Caldarelli, John S. Coon, *Tumour Angiogenesis and p53 Mutations. Prognosis in Head and Neck Cancer.* Arch. Otolaryngology Head Neck Surg. 1998; 124(1): 80–85

[335] Hamelin, R., Laurent-Puig, P., Olschwang, S., Jego, N., Asselain, B., Remvikos, Y., Girodet, J., Salmon, R.J., Thomas, G., *Association of p53 mutations with short survival in colorectal cancer.* Gastroenterology 1994; 106(1): 42–48

[336] T.C. Greiner, M.J. Moynihan, W.C. Chan, D.M. Lytle, A. Pedersen, J.R. Anderson, D.D. Weisenburger, *p53 mutations in mantle cell lymphoma are associated with variant cytology and predict a poor prognosis.* Blood 1996; 87(10): 4302–4310

[337] Wattle, E., Preudhomme, C., Hecquet, B., Vanrumbeke, M., Quesnel, B., Dervite, I., *p53 mutations are associated with resistance to chemotherapy and short survival in hematologic malignancies.* Blood 1994; 84: 3148–57

338 Wilson, W.H., Teruya-Feldstein, J., Fest, T., Harris, C., Steinburg, A.M., Jaffe, E.S. et al., *Relationship of p53, bcl2 and tumour proliferation to clinical drug resistance in non-Hodgkin's lymphomas.* Blood 1997; 89: 601–9

339 Kovach, J.S., Hartmann, A., Blaszyk, H., Cunningham, J., Schaid, D., Sommer, S.S., *Mutation detected by highly sensitive methods indicates that p53 gene mutations in breast cancer can have important prognostic value.* Proc. Natl. Acad. Sci. USA 1996; 93: 1029–34

340 Clahsen, P.C., Van de Velde, C.J., Duval, C., Pallud, C., Mandard, A.M., Delobelle, D.A. et al., *p53 protein accumulation and response to adjuvant chemotherapy in premenopausal women with node-negative early breast cancer.* J. Clin. Oncol. 1998; 16: 121–7

341 Matoba, S., Kang, J.G., Patino, W.D., Wragg, A., Boehm, M., Gavrilova, O., Hurley, P.J., Bunz, F. and Hwang, P.M., *p53 regulates mitochondrial respiration.* Science 2006; 312(5780): 1650–3

342 Dihua Yu, Bolin Liu, Tong Jing, Dantong Sun, Janet E. Price, S. Eva Singletary, Nuhad Ibrahim, Gabriel N. Hortobagyi, Mien-Chie Hung, *Overexpression of both p185$^{c-erbB2}$ and p170^{mdr-1} renders breast cancer cells highly resistant to taxol.* Oncogene 1998; 16(16): 2087–2094

343 Tan, M., Yu, D., *Molecular mechanisms of erbB2-mediated breast cancer chemoresistance.* Adv. Exp. Med. Biol. 2007; 608: 119–29

344 Daren Sh, Gongping He, Shilong Ca, Wensheng Pa, Hua-Zhong Zhan, Dihua Yu, Mien-Chie Hung, *Overexpression of the c-erbB-2/neu–encoded p185 protein in primary lung cancer.* Molecular Carcinogenesis1992; 5(3): 213–218

345 Shi, D., He, G., Cao, S., Pan, W., Zhang, H.Z., Yu, D., Hung, M.C., *Overexpression of the c-erbB-2/neu-encoded p185 protein in primary lung cancer.* Mol. Carcinog. 1992; 5(3): 213–8

346 Santin, A.D., Bellone, S., Roman, J.J., McKenney, J.K., Pecorelli, S., *Trastuzumab treatment in patients with advanced or recurrent endometrial carcinoma overexpressing HER2/neu.* Int. J. Gynaecol. Obstet. 2008; 102(2): 128–31

347 Iman Osman, Howard I. Scher, Marija Drobnjak, David Verbel, Michael Morris, David Agus, Jeffrey S. Ross, Carlos Cordon-Cardo. *HER-2/neu (p185neu) Protein Expression in the Natural or Treated History of Prostate Cancer.* Clin. Cancer Res. 2001; 7: 2643

348 S. Kapitanovic, S. Radosevic, M. Kapitanovic, S. Andelinovic, Z. Ferencic, M. Tavassoli, D. Primorac, Z. Sonicki, S. Spaventi, K. Pavelic, R. Spaventi, *The expression of p185(HER-2/neu) correlates with the stage of disease and survival in colorectal cancer.* Gastroenterology 1997; 112(4): 1103–13

349 Nanni, P., Pupa, S.M., Nicoletti, G., De Giovanni, C., Landuzzi, L., Rossi, I., Astolfi, A., Ricci, C., De Vecchi, R., Invernizzi, A.M., Di Carlo, E., Musiani, P., Forni, G., Menard, S., Lollini, P.L., *p185(neu) protein is required for tumour and anchorage-independent growth, not for cell proliferation of transgenic mammary carcinoma.* Int. J. Cancer 2000; 15; 87(2)186–94

350 Dalifard, I., Daver, A., Goussard, J., Lorimier, G., Gosse-Brun, S., Lortholary, A., Larra, F., *p185 overexpression in 220 samples of breast cancer undergoing primary surgery: comparison with c-erbB-2 gene amplification.* Int. J. Mol. Med. 1998; 1(5): 855–61

351 David B. Cook, Abdul A. Bustamam, Ian Brotherick, Brian K. Shenton, Colin H. Self, *Lectin ELISA for the c-erb-B2 Tumour Marker Protein p185 in Patients with Breast Cancer and Controls.* Clin. Chem. 1999; 45(2): 292–295

352 Oltvai, Z.N., Milliman, C.L. and Korsmeyer, S.J., *Bcl-2 Heterodimerizes In Vivo with a Conserved Homolog, Bax, That Accelerates Programed Cell Death.* Cell 1993; 74(4): 609–619

353 Wolter, K.G., Hsu, Y., Smith, C.L., Mechushtan, A., Xi, X. and Youle, R.J., *Movement of BAX from Cytosol to Mitochondria during Apoptosis.* J. Cell Biology 1997; 139 (5): 1281–1292

354 Estelle Schmitt, Alain Steyaert, Guido Cimoli and Richard Bertrand, *Bax-alpha promotes apoptosis induced by cancer chemotherapy and accelerates the activation of caspase 3-like cysteine proteases in p53 double mutant B lymphoma Namalwa cells.* Cell Death and Differentiation 1998; 5(6): 506–516

355 Miyashita, T., Krajewski, S., Krajewska, M., Wang, H.G., Lin, H.K., Liebermann, D.A., Hoffman, B., Reed, J.C., *Tumour suppressor p53 is a regulator of bcl-2 and bax gene expression in vitro and in vivo.* Oncogene 1994; 9(6): 1799–1805

356 Porebska, I., Wyrodek, E., Kosacka, M., Adamiak, J., Jankowska, R., Harłozińska-Szmyrka, A., *Apoptotic markers p53, Bcl-2 and Bax in primary lung cancer.* in vivo 2006; 20(5): 599–604

357 Li Yan Khor, Jennifer Moughan, Tahseen Al-Saleem, Elizabeth H. Hammond, Varagur Venkatesan, Seth A. Rosenthal, Mark A. Ritter, Howard M. Sandler, Gerald E. Hanks, William U. Shipley, Alan Pollack, *Bcl-2 and Bax Expression Predict Prostate Cancer Outcome in Men Treated with Androgen Deprivation and Radiotherapy on Radiation Therapy Oncology Group Protocol 92-02.* Clin. Cancer Res. 2007; 13: 3585

358 Hirofumi Yamamoto, Chew Yee Ngan and Morito Monden, *Cancer cells survive with survivin.* Cancer Sci. 2008; 99: 1709–1714

359 Tamm, I., Wang, Y., Sausville, E., Scudiero, D.A., Vigna, N., Oltersdorf, T., Reed, J.C., *IAP-family protein survivin inhibits caspase activity and apoptosis induced by Fas (CD95), Bax caspases, and anticancer drugs.* Cancer Res. 1998; 58(23): 5315–20

360 Grazia Ambrosini, Colette Adida and Dario C. Altieri, *A novel anti-apoptosis gene, survivin, expressed in cancer and lymphoma.* Nature Medicine 1997; 3: 917–921

361 Hemat, R.A.S., *Orthomolecularism, Principles and Practice.* Authorhouse, 2004

362 Masatsugu Ueda et al., *Survivin Gene Expression in Endometriosis.* J. Clinical Endocrinology & Metabolism 2002; 87(7): 3452–3459

363 Whitney Salz et al., *A Survivin Gene Signature Predicts Aggressive Tumour Behaviour.* Cancer Research 2005; 65: 3531–3534

364 Mirza, A., McGuirk, M., Hockenberry, T.N., Wu, Q., Ashar, H., Black, S., Wen, S.F., Wang, L., Kirschmeier, P., Bishop, W.R., Nielsen, L.L., Pickett, C.B., Liu, S., *Human survivin is negatively regulated by wild-type p53 and participates in p53-dependent apoptotic pathway.* Oncogene 2002; 21(17): 2613–22

365 Salz, W. et al., *A survivin gene signature predicts aggressive tumour behaviour.* Urologic Oncology: Seminars and Original Investigations 2005; 24(6): 563–564

366 McDougall, S.R, Anderson, A.R.A., Chaplain, M.A.J., *Mathematical modelling of dynamic adaptive tumour-induced angiogenesis: Clinical implications and therapeutic targeting strategies.* J. Theoretical Biol. 2006; 241(3): 564–589

367 Prior, B.M., Yang, H.T., Terjung, R.L., *What makes vessels grow with exercise training?* J. Applied Physiol. 2004; 97(3): 1119–28

368 Bergers, G., Benjamin, L.E., *Tumourigenesis and the angiogenic switch. Nature Reviews.* Cancer 2003; 3(6): 401–10

369 Hanahan, D., Weinberg, R.A., *The hallmarks of cancer.* Cell 2000; 100: 57–70

370 Hanahan, D., Weinberg, R.A., *Hallmarks of cancer: the next generation.* Cell 2011; 144(5): 646–74

371 Beard, J., *The Enzyme Treatment of Cancer.* London: Chatto and Windus, 1911

372 P. Biava, *Cancer and the Search for Lost Meaning.* North Atlantic Books, 2009

373 Yoshida, B.A., Sokoloff, M.M., Welch, D.R., Rinker-Schaeffer, C.W., *Metastasis-suppressor genes: a review and perspective on an emerging field.* J. Natl. Cancer Inst. 2000; 92(21): 1717–30

374 Prior, B.M., Yang, H.T., Terjung, R.L., *What makes vessels grow with exercise training?* J. Applied Physiol. 2004; 97 (3): 1119–28

375 Navarro, M., *72nd Science Meeting of the Cavite Med. Soc.* 1959; Trece Martires City, Philippines

376 Glenn Drano, *Cytokines in cancer pathogenesis and cancer therapy.* Nature Reviews Cancer 2004; 4: 11–22

[377] Escárcega, R.O., Fuentes-Alexandro, S., García-Carrasco, M., Gatica, A., Zamora, A., *The transcription factor nuclear factor-κB and cancer.* Clinical Oncology (Royal College of Radiologists (Great Britain)) 2007; 19 (2): 154–61 doi:10.1016/j.clon.2006.11.013. PMID 17355113

[378] Liu, F., Bardhan, K., Yang, D., Thangaraju, M., Ganapathy, V., Liles, G., Lee, J., Liu, K., *F-κB directly regulates Fas transcription to modulate Fas-mediated apoptosis and tumour suppression.* J. Biol. Chem. 2012; doi:10.1074/jbc.M112.356279. PMID 22669972.

INDEX

Figures in **bold** signify a section dedicated to the subject.

PRINTED AND BOUND BY:

Copytech (UK) Limited trading as Printondemand-worldwide,
9 Culley Court, Bakewell Road, Orton Southgate. Peterborough,
PE2 6XD, United Kingdom.